THE PROMISES AND PERILS OF DIGITAL STRATEGIES IN ACHIEVING HEALTH EQUITY

Workshop Summary

Karen M. Anderson and Steve Olson, *Rapporteurs*

Roundtable on the Promotion of Health Equity
and the Elimination of Health Disparities

Board on Population Health and Public Health Practice

Health and Medicine Division

The National Academies of
SCIENCES • ENGINEERING • MEDICINE

THE NATIONAL ACADEMIES PRESS
Washington, DC
www.nap.edu

THE NATIONAL ACADEMIES PRESS   500 Fifth Street, NW   Washington, DC 20001

This activity was supported by contracts between the National Academy of Sciences and the Aetna Foundation, The Kresge Foundation (245367), Merck & Co., Inc. (APA-2013-1223), the U.S. Department of Health and Human Services [Centers for Disease Control and Prevention] (200-2011-38807, TO#34), and the U.S. Department of Health and Human Services [Health Resources and Services Administration] (HHSH25034010T). Any opinions, findings, conclusions, or recommendations expressed in this publication do not necessarily reflect the views of any organization or agency that provided support for the project.

International Standard Book Number-13:   978-0-309-43891-9
International Standard Book Number-10:   0-309-43891-8
Digit Object Identifier: 10.17226/23439

Additional copies of this report are available for sale from the National Academies Press, 500 Fifth Street, NW, Keck 360, Washington, DC 20001; (800) 624-6242 or (202) 334-3313; http://www.nap.edu.

Copyright 2016 by the National Academy of Sciences. All rights reserved.

Printed in the United States of America

Suggested citation: National Academies of Sciences, Engineering, and Medicine. 2016. *The promises and perils of digital strategies in achieving health equity: Workshop summary.* Washington, DC: The National Academies Press. doi: 10.17226/23439.

The National Academies of
SCIENCES · ENGINEERING · MEDICINE

The **National Academy of Sciences** was established in 1863 by an Act of Congress, signed by President Lincoln, as a private, nongovernmental institution to advise the nation on issues related to science and technology. Members are elected by their peers for outstanding contributions to research. Dr. Ralph J. Cicerone is president.

The **National Academy of Engineering** was established in 1964 under the charter of the National Academy of Sciences to bring the practices of engineering to advising the nation. Members are elected by their peers for extraordinary contributions to engineering. Dr. C. D. Mote, Jr., is president.

The **National Academy of Medicine** (formerly the Institute of Medicine) was established in 1970 under the charter of the National Academy of Sciences to advise the nation on medical and health issues. Members are elected by their peers for distinguished contributions to medicine and health. Dr. Victor J. Dzau is president.

The three Academies work together as the **National Academies of Sciences, Engineering, and Medicine** to provide independent, objective analysis and advice to the nation and conduct other activities to solve complex problems and inform public policy decisions. The Academies also encourage education and research, recognize outstanding contributions to knowledge, and increase public understanding in matters of science, engineering, and medicine.

Learn more about the National Academies of Sciences, Engineering, and Medicine at **www.national-academies.org**.

PLANNING COMMITTEE ON THE PROMISES AND PERILS OF DIGITAL STRATEGIES IN ACHIEVING HEALTH EQUITY[1]

GILLIAN BARCLAY (*Co-Chair*), Aetna Foundation
ANTONIA M. VILLARRUEL (*Co-Chair*), University of Pennsylvania
CAROLINE McKAY, U.S. Outcomes Research, Merck
MELISSA SIMON, Northwestern University
ROHIT VARMA, University of Southern California

---

[1] The National Academies of Sciences, Engineering, and Medicine's planning committees are solely responsible for organizing the workshop, identifying topics, and choosing speakers. The responsibility for the published workshop summary rests with the workshop rapporteurs and the institution.

ROUNDTABLE ON THE PROMOTION OF HEALTH EQUITY AND THE ELIMINATION OF HEALTH DISPARITIES[1]

MILDRED THOMPSON (*Co-Chair*), PolicyLink
ANTONIA M. VILLARRUEL (*Co-Chair*), University of Pennsylvania
PATRICIA BAKER, Connecticut Health Foundation
GILLIAN BARCLAY, Aetna Foundation
ANNE C. BEAL, Patient-Centered Outcomes Research Institute
NED CALONGE, The Colorado Trust
IRENE DANKWA-MULLAN, National Institutes of Health
JAMILA DAVISON, ACM Medical Transition Care
FRANCISCO GARCIA, Pima County Department of Health
ALLAN GOLDBERG, Merck & Co., Inc.
J. NADINE GRACIA, U.S. Department of Health and Human Services
JEFFREY A. HENDERSON, Black Hills Center for American Indian Health
EVE J. HIGGINBOTHAM, University of Pennsylvania
CARA V. JAMES, Centers for Medicare & Medicaid Services
OCTAVIO MARTINEZ, Hogg Foundation for Mental Health
NEWELL McELWEE, Merck & Co., Inc.
PHYLLIS W. MEADOWS, The Kresge Foundation
AMELIE G. RAMIREZ, University of Texas Health Science Center
MELISSA SIMON, Northwestern University Feinberg School of Medicine
CHRISTINE TORBERT, Health Resources and Services Administration
PATTIE TUCKER, Centers for Disease Control and Prevention
ROHIT VARMA, University of Illinois–Chicago
WINSTON F. WONG, Kaiser Permanente
TERRI D. WRIGHT, American Public Health Association

HMD Staff

KAREN M. ANDERSON, Senior Program Officer
COLIN FINK, Senior Program Assistant
ROSE MARIE MARTINEZ, Senior Board Director
ANNA MARTIN, Senior Program Assistant

---

[1] The National Academies of Sciences, Engineering, and Medicine's forums and roundtables do not issue, review, or approve individual documents. The responsibility for the published workshop summary rests with the workshop rapporteurs and the institution.

Reviewers

This workshop summary has been reviewed in draft form by individuals chosen for their diverse perspectives and technical expertise. The purpose of this independent review is to provide candid and critical comments that will assist the institution in making its published workshop summary as sound as possible and to ensure that the workshop summary meets institutional standards for objectivity, evidence, and responsiveness to the study charge. The review comments and draft manuscript remain confidential to protect the integrity of the process. We wish to thank the following individuals for their review of this workshop summary:

Gillian Christie, The Vitality Institute
Chazeman S. Jackson, U.S. Department of Health and Human Services
Elizabeth Ofili, Morehouse School of Medicine
Pattie Tucker, Centers for Disease Control and Prevention

Although the reviewers listed above have provided many constructive comments and suggestions, they did not see the final draft of the workshop summary before its release. The review of this workshop summary was overseen by **Derek Yach,** The Vitality Group. He was responsible for making certain that an independent examination of this workshop summary was carried out in accordance with institutional procedures and that all review comments were carefully considered. Responsibility for the final content of this workshop summary rests entirely with the rapporteurs and the institution.

Contents

ACRONYMS AND ABBREVIATIONS   xiii

1   **INTRODUCTION OF THE WORKSHOP**   1
Highlights of the Workshop, 3
Organization of the Report, 4

2   **TECHNOLOGY AND HEALTH DISPARITIES**   5
Equity at the Henry Ford Health System, 6
The Potential of Technology, 7
The Perils of Technology, 8
Engaging Communities, 9
The Diversity of Hope, 11
Realizing the Promise of Mobile Technologies, 11
Mobile Technologies and Health Disparities, 12
Using Mobile Technologies to Change Behavior, 13

3   **ENGAGING PROVIDERS AND RACIAL/ETHNIC MINORITY PATIENTS IN DIGITAL STRATEGIES**   15
Creating a Movement for Change, 16
The Value of Theories, 18
A Health Literacy Perspective on Health Disparities, 19
Designing Systems for Health Literacy and Equity, 22

4 **EXAMPLES OF ENGAGING RACIAL/ETHNIC MINORITY
   COMMUNITIES IN DIGITAL HEALTH STRATEGIES**   27
   Reducing Digital and Health Inequities in Latina Immigrant
      Communities, 28
   A Tailored Web-Based Intervention for Young MSM in
      Southeast Michigan, 30

5 **POLICY AND TECHNOLOGY PERSPECTIVES**   35
   Top-Down and Bottom-Up Approaches to Policy, 36
   The Policy Perspective from an Integrated Health Care Delivery
      System, 38
   Observations from a Technology Developer, 41

6 **SYNTHESIS OF WORKSHOP MESSAGES**   43
   Generating Evidence of Effectiveness, 43
   Privacy and Sustainability, 44
   The In-Person Component, 44
   Involving Communities, 45
   Scalability and Adaptability, 46
   Involving Providers, 46

REFERENCES   47

APPENDIXES

A EXAMPLES OF EHEALTH SOLUTIONS FEATURED
   AT THE WORKSHOP   49
B WORKSHOP AGENDA   57
C SPEAKER BIOGRAPHICAL SKETCHES   61

Acronyms and Abbreviations

ACA	Affordable Care Act
CBPR	community-based participatory research
CHESS	Community Health Engagement Survey Solutions
EHR	electronic health record
GIS	geographic information system
HARC	HIV/AIDS Resource Center
HIPAA	Health Insurance Portability and Accountability Act
HITECH	Health Information Technology for Economic and Clinical Health
HIV/STI	human immunodeficiency virus/sexually transmitted illness
ICD	*International Statistical Classification of Diseases and Related Health Problems*
IOM	Institute of Medicine
IPV	interpersonal partner violence
LGBTQ	lesbian, gay, bisexual, transgender, queer
m(Dad)	Mobile Dad

MSM	men who have sex with men
MVP	moderate to vigorous physical activity
NIH	National Institutes of Health
NSF	National Science Foundation
PHR	personal health record
SNAP	Supplemental Nutrition Assistant Program
WIN	Women-Inspired Neighborhood
YMSM	young men who have sex with men

1

Introduction of the Workshop[1]

Health care is in the midst of a dramatic transformation in the United States. Spurred by technological advances, economic imperatives, and governmental policies, information technologies are rapidly being applied to health care in an effort to improve access, enhance quality, and decrease costs. At the same time, the use of technologies by the consumers of health care is changing how people interact with the health care system and with health information.

These changes in health care have the potential both to exacerbate and to diminish the stark disparities in health and well-being that exist among population groups in the United States. If the benefits of technology flow disproportionately to those who already enjoy better coverage, use, and outcomes than disadvantaged groups, health disparities could increase. But if technologies can be developed and implemented in such a way as to improve access and enhance quality for the members of all groups, the ongoing transformation of health care could reduce the gaps among groups while improving health care for all. As a recent report from the Institute of Medicine (IOM) stated, "Facilitating patient and population contribution to, and control of, their health information has the potential to provide fur-

---

[1] The planning committee's role was limited to planning the workshop, and the workshop summary has been prepared by the rapporteurs as a factual account of what occurred at the workshop. Statements, recommendations, and opinions expressed are those of the individual presenters and participants and are not necessarily endorsed or verified by the National Academies of Sciences, Engineering, and Medicine. They should not be construed as reflecting any group consensus.

ther insights into, and opportunities to address, disparities in underserved populations" (IOM, 2011, p. 38).

To explore this potential, the National Academies of Sciences, Engineering, and Medicine's Roundtable on the Promotion of Health Equity and the Elimination of Health Disparities held a workshop at Wayne State University on October 2, 2014. The focus of the workshop was on (1) how communities are using digital health technologies[2] to improve health outcomes for racial and ethnic minority populations, (2) how community engagement can improve access to high-quality health information for members of these groups, and (3) models of successful technology-based strategies to reduce health disparities. Box 1-1 lists the goals of the workshop.

The workshop was held in Detroit, Michigan, on the campus of Wayne State University, to emphasize both the promises and the perils cited in the workshop's title. Detroit has some of the worst health disparities in the nation, yet it is also at the center of work on reducing these disparities, noted M. Roy Wilson, the president of Wayne State University and a former official at the National Institutes of Health (NIH) in charge of the NIH health disparities research agenda. Wayne State University has the only NIH perinatal research branch outside of the NIH campus in Bethesda, Maryland, partly because of the high infant mortality rate in the city (discussed in more detail in Chapter 2). Wayne State also has been a leader in other areas related to health disparities. The Barbara Ann Karmanos Cancer Institute has been looking at the determinants of health among survivors of cancer who have access to the Internet and those who do not. A research project in the medical school is looking at the effect of text message reminders about adherence to blood pressure medication. An interdisciplinary team has developed a sensor that includes a heart monitor and a Bluetooth connection to a smartphone to identify potentially dangerous heart rate increases. "We are very proud of everything that is going on here," said Wilson.

This report provides a summary of the presentations at the workshop and the discussions that occurred among workshop participants. (Comments made by presenters during the discussion sessions generally are included in the summaries of their talks.) The observations made in the report are of the workshop as a whole and should not be seen as the conclusions of the workshop participants, the Roundtable on the Promotion of Health Equity and the Elimination of Health Disparities, or the Academies. However, they provide many valuable insights into future steps that could be taken to reduce health disparities in the United States.

---

[2] For the purposes of this workshop, "digital health technologies" encompasses all types of personal technology. However, the majority of the technologies described in this summary are cell phone based or interactive websites.

> **BOX 1-1**
> **Goals of the Workshop**
>
> - Discuss the opportunities to use digital health technologies as a population health strategy to reduce health disparities and promote health equity in the United States.
> - Explore how racial and ethnic minority populations and communities in the United States can be engaged in efforts that use digital health strategies to reduce racial and ethnic health disparities.
> - Develop effective strategies that engage racial and ethnic minority populations and communities in using digital health strategies to reduce health disparities.
> - Explore the different types of digital health technologies used in efforts to reduce health disparities and promote health equity in the United States.
> - Highlight examples of digital health strategies designed to reduce health disparities and promote health equity in the United States.

HIGHLIGHTS OF THE WORKSHOP

In the final session of the workshop, Gillian Barclay, vice president of the Aetna Foundation, summarized some of the main messages that she heard during the presentations and discussions. The following draws on Barclay's remarks and on comments made over the course of the day to identify the major ideas that arose during the workshop:

- The main point gleaned from the workshop, said Barclay, is that technology "is really all about people." Addressing racial and ethnic health disparities and increasing health equity in the United States "goes back to the foundation of placing people first and not technology first," she said.
- Community engagement is essential in designing, evaluating, and adapting technology-based interventions aimed at improving health in racial and ethnic minority groups.
- Reducing health disparities requires going beyond both the use of technology and health care in general to a "health-in-all-policies" approach. Education, transportation, and other sectors can all contribute to the reduction of disparities.
- Systems and patterns are major determinants of health disparities. Looking at the potential of technology to reduce health disparities requires consideration of these systems and patterns, not just particular events.

ORGANIZATION OF THE REPORT

Following this introduction to the report, Chapter 2 summarizes the remarks of the two keynote presenters at the workshop, both of whom provided overarching views of health disparities and technology issues on local, regional, and national levels.

Chapter 3 examines a wide range of issues associated with the use of technology to reduce health disparities, including health literacy, community engagement, and the role of theory in program development. Chapter 4 looks in greater detail at two specific programs as a way of exploring how these issues play out in practice.

Chapter 5 considers the broader policy and technology issues that shape health equity initiatives. In Chapter 6, two respondents identified the key messages emerging from the presentations and discussions at the workshop.

Appendix A provides descriptions of nine programs that workshop participants learned about during a "virtual poster session" at lunch. Appendix B contains the workshop agenda and Appendix C gives biographies of the speakers at the workshop.

2

Technology and Health Disparities

Important Points Highlighted by the Speakers

- The tremendous expansion in the use of technology provides many opportunities to work with communities to reduce health disparities. (Nilsen, Wisdom)
- In particular, mobile technologies have a unique potential to reduce disparities because of their extensive use in racial and ethnic minority communities. (Nilsen, Wisdom)
- As just one example, a community online campaign in the city of Detroit has substantially reduced the infant mortality rate in targeted communities. (Wisdom)
- The use of technology can be resisted if it does not produce benefits that outweigh the time and efforts its use entails. (Nilsen)
- Community engagement can help shape interventions that effectively address the needs of the community. (Nilsen, Wisdom)

Globally, more people own a mobile phone than own a toothbrush, noted Kimberlydawn Wisdom, senior vice president of community health and equity and chief wellness and diversity officer in the Henry Ford Health System, in her opening keynote address at the conference. Seventy-seven percent of U.S. seniors own a cell phone or smartphone. By 2020, a projected 200 billion smart devices will communicate through wireless technologies—the equivalent of 26 devices for every person on the planet (Cisco, 2015). Already, 42 percent of U.S. hospitals are using digital health technology to treat patients, and technology use is growing "at an exponential pace," said Wisdom.

EQUITY AT THE HENRY FORD HEALTH SYSTEM

The Henry Ford Health System, which was founded by Henry Ford in 1915 and has five hospitals in southeastern Michigan, has a major focus on the elimination of health and health care disparities, said Wisdom. Its vision statement is "transforming lives and communities through health and wellness—one person at a time," and one of the seven pillars upholding that mission is community. The system has pursued its goal of health and health care equity through grant funding and system support, but support for the mission also has been personal. Wisdom recounted an episode when she wanted to publish a paper showing that African Americans were having poorer outcomes related to diabetes care than their Caucasian counterparts in the health plan. She received the full support of the system's chief executive officer to do so. "I cannot underscore that enough, because having individuals like that who will say, 'Do the thing that is right, even though it may not reflect perfectly favorably on the organization,' shows that we are paying attention to these things," Wisdom said.

She also described an initiative from the 1990s in which the Detroit Piston's basketball player Joe Dumars participated in what was called the African American Initiative for Male Health Improvement. "As we talk about eliminating disparities, you need to somehow find the route that is going to be most culturally appropriate to get the change that you need," Wisdom explained.

The Institute of Medicine report *Unequal Treatment: Confronting Racial and Ethnic Disparities in Health Care* (IOM, 2002) provided tremendous momentum by demonstrating "that the work we were doing was absolutely important and that those disparities were profound and persistent," said Wisdom. The *National Healthcare Disparities Report 2012* (AHRQ, 2013) likewise drew attention to what Wisdom was seeing in the clinic: vast differences in care and in outcomes for people of color versus the white population.

When Wisdom returned to the Henry Ford Health System after serving as surgeon general for the State of Michigan, she inserted into her terms for returning that health disparities be integrated into the results presented to the board. That led to the launch in 2009 of a health care equity campaign with the goal of increasing "knowledge, awareness, and opportunities to ensure that health care equity is understood and practiced by Henry Ford providers and other staff, the research community, and the community at large."[1]

---

[1] More information about the campaign is available at http://www.henryford.com/healthcare equitycampaign (accessed May 18, 2016).

THE POTENTIAL OF TECHNOLOGY

The Henry Ford Health System has been working directly with communities to eliminate the causes of disparities. For example, it launched a LiveWell Center of Excellence, which involved the development of a strategic plan, the launch of a new website (HenryFordLiveWell.com), and the convening of a childhood obesity prevention initiative. It also has worked with thousands of young people in the community to drive environmental and behavioral change.

Technology has played a greater and greater role in these efforts, Wisdom observed. For example, young people use technology extensively, so the task with them has been to use technology as a tool to advance the system's message—including working with a local rapper to develop a health-promoting song that was posted on YouTube.

The Henry Ford Health System also has been using a variety of technologies to communicate with and monitor patients remotely to improve health outcomes. Electronic medicine-dispensing systems can reduce the risk of medication mismanagement. Telehealth systems can help patients with chronic disease manage their own care and help prevent visits to emergency rooms and hospitalizations.

With the Partnership for a Healthier America led by First Lady Michelle Obama, the system has joined in the Healthy Hospital Food Commitment, which includes a third-party vendor that audits compliance.[2] The commitment includes a smartphone app that builds menus, provides complete nutrition information, offers other healthy living tools, and supports the 5-2-1-0 message (targeted at children), which stands for consumption of 5 or more fruits and vegetables per day, 2 hours or less of recreational screen time, 1 hour of physical activity, and 0 sugar-sweetened beverages. "We know that many disparities exist around diabetes related to weight," said Wisdom, adding "We are trying to find ways to use technology to engage young people and their families."

The Henry Ford Health System also has been working with three other major health systems in the area to address the infant mortality challenge. As Wisdom noted, in the city of Detroit, an average of about 200 babies die per year. "It is astounding that you could be here with these four mega-health-systems, [and] with the NIH perinatal branch right here, and yet we see these appallingly high infant mortality rates," she said. In a collaborative effort, the four health systems have come together as leaders, funders, strategists, communicators, and implementers to address these and other disparities.

---

[2] The third-party audit is conducted by the Altarum Institute, Center for Active Design, Food & Nutrition Policy Consultants LLC, RTI International, and the Rudd Center for Food Policy and Obesity.

As part of its effort to eliminate infant mortality, the system has received a grant from the W.K. Kellogg Foundation to use social media to inspire change through the Women-Inspired Neighborhood (WIN) network. A recently launched website (www.WINnetworkDetroit.org) seeks to empower not just low-income pregnant women but women of reproductive age, mothers, and caregivers—"the grandmothers and the aunts and the sisters," said Wisdom. The network is active on Facebook, Instagram, Twitter, and blogs. "If we are going to address disparities, we are going to have to reach people in the model and medium in which they are most comfortable."

In three neighborhoods with high infant mortality where the network is active, more than 200 women have delivered without an infant death. "[We have] driven the infant mortality rate to zero. We are really pleased with that," Wisdom explained.[3]

One interesting observation has been that a major contributor to infant mortality is social isolation. "You would think, with all this technology, how could people experience social isolation? But there is a tremendous amount of people feeling disconnected," she said. In response, the network has been developing ways to hold virtual sessions with women to teach and reassure them even when it is difficult for them to travel.

THE PERILS OF TECHNOLOGY

Technology is a "tremendous tool," said Wisdom, but it also has potential perils. As an example, Wisdom cited the recent effort to collect data about race, ethnicity, and primary language at a detailed level. To develop a common platform, the system borrowed a tool developed by the Robert Wood Johnson Foundation called We Ask Because We Care. However, collecting race, ethnicity, and primary language data "is a heavy lift at the point of service," which led to resistance from the frontline staff, she explained.

The use of the electronic health record (EHR) to reduce disparities is another example of potential difficulties. "Many individuals, whether it is meaningful use or in other arenas, have access to the technology, but using it in a way that can truly improve outcomes and close the health disparities gap is a major issue," said Wisdom. With EHRs, providers can have their "faces glued to a screen," giving them less time to interact personally with patients, adding that "it is great to have this technology, but if it limits that face-to-face time, if it limits the ability to really understand and communicate well to patients, it could have an unintended consequence."

In addition, the Henry Ford Health System uses a tool known as MyChart to give patients access to their medical record. But surveys have

---

[3] The previous infant mortality rate was 15 deaths per 1,000 births.

shown that only about 12 percent of adults in the system have proficient health literacy—defined as a patient's ability to obtain, understand, and act on health information—which has consequences in terms of patient use of health information. (Health literacy is discussed in more detail in the next chapter.) Wisdom noted, "One of the things that worries me is that, as we try to close the digital divide, unintended consequences of widening the divide in terms of outcomes could be an issue."

Additional challenges include

- evaluating tools like MyChart to ensure that different racial/ethnic population subgroups are using it at the same rate,
- the potential loss of personal interactions as technology becomes more prominent in health care, and
- making the data accessible in communities.

Real-time data are important to eliminate disparities, because much of the public health data related to disparities are dated, said Wisdom, adding, "We need to be able to understand, in real time, what the data show, as well as communicate that to the community, so they can become partners in helping us eliminate health and health care disparities."

ENGAGING COMMUNITIES

As was discussed throughout the workshop, community engagement has been a key component of the Henry Ford Health System's efforts. For example, the system has used community-based participatory research to bring audiences to the table, where their voices can be heard while initiatives are being planned. Focus groups are another way to involve communities, although Wisdom said that communities need to be involved in meetings in an ongoing way.

> On our evaluation team for our WIN Network Detroit, we had a community health worker at every single meeting [who provided] invaluable information. For instance, we were saying how do we incentivize our target women to do certain things. She said a lot of the women are having case workers come to their home because they want child protective services and people coming to review their home setting, what they are doing, and how they are evolving as mothers and caretakers. They said having them go through a class and giving them a certificate to show their caseworker would be of tremendous value. That is better than a $5 or $10 gift certificate to go buy something at Target. Give them a certificate to show that they are meeting the requirements in order to protect their children and keep their families. That kind of information—I would have never come up with that.

Many of the community health workers are from the neighborhoods they (the community health workers) are serving. The women with whom they work see them as best friends. "They are my aunt. They are my confidante. . . . For the medical community, we want the data. We want all the hard stuff. [But] those relationships are key. They share information that they ordinarily would not share with their provider," Wisdom explained.

Community health workers are directly involved in the research and outreach being done by the system. They have been included in abstracts presented at national meetings. One community health worker spoke at the American Public Health Association meeting and "had the room in tears," according to Wisdom, adding, "She did a much better job than I did in terms of engaging the audience."

People who are not traditional health care professionals also need to be empowered, she said. For example, when students learn about healthy eating, they can be ambassadors to their peers. "In many ways, they are our secret weapon, because . . . other students in their class will listen a lot better to them, particularly when they are in the lunch line, than they will to somebody coming in with a white coat saying you ought to do this," she said. The system also has been examining technology that can help people learn through games, and it is very interested in mobile applications that are patient centered and easily accessible, even for patients who are not highly health literate.

A researcher at the Henry Ford Health System recently received a Patient-Centered Outcomes Research Institute grant to pursue patient engagement and patient-driven research in an effort to increase dissemination and implementation. The objectives are to understand the choices patients face, to align research questions and methods with patient needs, and to provide patients and clinicians with information for better processes and decisions. "We are going to learn a lot in that process," said Wisdom.

The Henry Ford Health System is collaborating with more than 40 leading nonprofit health care organizations to create a menu of proven community health practices that work "from the top of the mission statement to the bottom line," Wisdom observed. The objective is to show that there is an economic case around eliminating health and health care disparities. Another objective is to make technology the servant and not the master of the vision, in part by developing specifications and a framework for the development and acquisition of information technology that forms a single integrated system for clinical and community settings.

THE DIVERSITY OF HOPE

The world will look much different in 5 years as technologies develop and as policies and laws such as the Affordable Care Act continue to be implemented, Wisdom said. Health care will be much more patient and community centered, with health care professionals supporting the efforts of individuals. "It is going to become very exciting," she noted.

Individual habits also can change. For example, Wisdom pointed to the spreading idea that sitting is the new smoking, adding that "I envision a future where at meetings like this people will be standing and walking even 2 miles an hour on some kind of device. . . . If you have gone to your meetings for the day, you will have gotten your 10,000 or 20,000 steps in because you have been in meetings all day." At Henry Ford Health System, for example, some meetings are done while walking around the building.

Winston closed by showing a mural that is composed of many hundreds of individual drawings submitted by people in the community. Each small tile in the mural represents the artwork of someone who was asked to envision the future, and contributors can zoom in to their drawings on a special website. The mural[4] is being put on buildings in three neighborhoods in Detroit "as a way to show that we are there and you have a voice and we want together to bring hope to the community," she concluded.

REALIZING THE PROMISE OF MOBILE TECHNOLOGIES

For much of the history of the computer age, computers have been tied to plugs, whether for power or for Internet access, which meant that some people could access and use computers while others could not, observed Wendy Nilsen, health scientist administrator at the Office of Behavioral and Social Sciences Research and program director for the Smart and Connected Health program at the National Science Foundation (NSF), in the second keynote address of the workshop. But now the world has gone mobile, and "Mobile is where we can finally reduce the digital divide," she began.

At the National Institutes of Health, *mHealth* refers to any wireless device carried by or on a person that accepts or transmits health data and information. Such devices include sensors, such as implantable miniature sensors and nanosensors, monitors such as wireless accelerometers and blood pressure and glucose monitors, and mobile phones and tablets.

Mobile technologies "can expand the things we care about in health to the real world instead of having it stay only in rarified academic centers,"

---

[4] An image of the mural is available in the speaker presentation by Kimberlydawn Wisdom, posted on the Roundtable website at: http://www.nationalacademies.org/hmd/Activities/SelectPops/HealthDisparities/2014-OCT-02.aspx (accessed May 18, 2016) and on the Project S.N.A.P. webpage: http://projectsnap.org/mural/winnetworkdetroit (accessed May 18, 2016).

said Nilsen. These technologies can generate user-friendly tools for enhancing health. They can change the questions people ask about their own health and about the information available to them. These technologies can scale up to entire populations, and they can facilitate more efficient and representative clinical trials. Nilsen discussed each of these topics in turn.

MOBILE TECHNOLOGIES AND HEALTH DISPARITIES

mHealth technologies can help reduce disparities in a variety of ways, Nilsen observed. First, they are used very widely. African Americans lead whites in their use of mobile phones, with Latinos only a few percentage points behind, and African Americans and Latinos lead whites in their use of mobile data applications. Those with less education and lower incomes use cell phones almost as much as others. Not everyone has access to mobile technologies all the time. Some people might lose coverage for a while, but they tend to get it back, Nilsen acknowledged.

According to national surveys, about two-thirds of cell phone owners find themselves checking their phone for messages, alerts, or calls even when they do not notice the phone vibrating or ringing. Nilsen cited a recent newspaper article saying that many people begin to panic when they cannot check their cell phone for 4 hours or more. "If you walk out the door this morning without your laptop, without your ID badge, you are going to keep going. You are going to figure out a way around it. If you walked out the door without your phone, are you going back?" she wondered.

Young adults are leading the way in the use of mobile data applications. They also are pioneering new ways of using mobile technologies—for example, by taking pictures of visible health problems and sending them to their health care providers. Older Americans still lag in their use of cell phones but increasing numbers are discovering the value of these technologies.

One great advantage of mobile technologies is the degree to which they can be customized by languages, applications, ringtones, and other features, including how they are decorated. These technologies are "intimate in a way that we have never had technology intimate before," said Nilsen.

Mobile technologies can centralize communication. They can be a health hub, transferring photos, to-do or to-ask lists, and messages among patients and a care team. They can provide patients with interventions and information programs alongside self-tracked information. Patients can ask questions when those questions occur to them, not in a rushed clinical encounter. Mobile technologies also could allow patients to respond to short and brief questionnaires rather than long forms. "Why can't we think the way industry has been thinking—getting a lot of information, constantly updated, but in the same way doing it simply?" Nilsen asked.

Finally, mobile technologies can greatly increase the representativeness of clinical research. Patient-generated data can be combined with clinical information, assessment data, and treatment plans to make what Nilsen called a "fabulous health stew." Technology could gather the information that is routinely gathered in doctors' offices, such as weight and blood pressure information, and it can collect such information in an ongoing way and not at one point. Very few patients ever go to academic medical centers, which tend to see only the most complex and hardest cases, yet this is where most research is carried out. Technologies could make it possible to do such research remotely, she said, adding, "We can have high touch when we need, but can we have tech touch the rest of the time, so people do not have to come to an academic center?"

USING MOBILE TECHNOLOGIES TO CHANGE BEHAVIOR

Mobile technologies are clearly changing behavior, said Nilsen, though not always for the better. "Think about what Madison Avenue is doing. They are using YouTube. They are using Twitter. They are using apps. They are using all of this to change behavior. Let us change it back. Let us get it the way we need it," she commented.

Mobile technologies provide opportunities for engagement that rival unhealthy competition, Nilsen said. Mobile technologies provide the potential to make healthy behaviors enjoyable and desirable. They can get people moving and eating better. They provide real-time information when and where people need it, and they are integrated into people's lives. "Think of how we can capture all that glitzy world that we never could touch in health," she said. For example, smartphones could tell when someone is at a fast food restaurant and suggest healthy options. Another example Nilsen mentioned is the iPeriod app, which allows women to track their menstrual cycles, adding "Why aren't we thinking about how you partner with iPeriod to make sure not only are you tracking your period, so you are not getting pregnant, but what are you doing about your diabetes, too?"

Sensors that collect information across populations and over time also can change behaviors. For example, body sensors being used by overweight young Latinas are being embraced by those who use them, she explained, adding, "These girls love to show off their sensors. . . . The moms said, 'We want to do it, too.'" Text messages can be designed for people to manage chronic diseases. Health care providers can intervene remotely with greater frequency than for traditional care, with real-time management and a reduction in acute care. People can use their technologies to have private or difficult questions answered, enabling a proactive, timely, person-centered approach to health care. Wireless sensors can connect with the electronic health record, providing information for predictive health assessment frameworks.

To reduce disparities, people need actionable data, said Nilsen, explaining, "It has to be good for something. It cannot just cause a liability. It has to be able to provide information to everybody that works." Communities also need to be integral to the planning effort, said Nilsen. "What I think would work does not matter. I am not the one it is going to target," she said. Only by spending lots of time talking with people, from high users to nonusers, is it possible to figure out what will work. "When they use their device, what kind of things would work for them? How would it work for them? That is when it is successful," she said.

One way to teach people about these approaches is to involve young people, who may not be formally trained but are intuitively good at using devices. In Nilsen's work, young people have become very involved. "I work at NSF, and one of the things that we find is [young people] are very interested in this area, even in high school, looking at how do you build an app, how do you build a program, how do you think about that," she said.

The missing link, said Nielsen in response to a question, is user-centered design—creating technologies, programs, and information that people want to use. Industry has much to teach health care about this issue, as do the users of technologies and communities as a whole. Technologies such as YouTube have been successful in capturing huge audiences. If such technologies could be directed to reducing health disparities, great progress could be made. People are using technology to change behavior, Nilsen concluded, adding, "You can too."

3

Engaging Providers and Racial/Ethnic Minority Patients in Digital Strategies

> **Important Points Highlighted by the Speakers**
>
> - Digital technologies have attributes that distinguish them from other interventions to reduce health disparities, including high rates of use in racial and ethnic minority communities. (Horn, Parker)
> - Greater communication between the developers and users of technology could reduce the disconnection between where digital strategies are developed and where the needs are greatest. (Horn, Norman, Parker)
> - The optimal use of technologies requires having good theories about why and where they work. (Norman, Parker, Pavel)
> - As people are overwhelmed by the amount and complexity of information they receive, they can be expected to question some of the systems enabled by digital technologies. (Parker)
> - Patients are the experts on their own health, which requires that health care systems find ways to engage patients more effectively. (Horn, Parker)

Four presentations at the workshop examined the broad issues that affect any effort to use technology to reduce health disparities. These issues range widely, from health literacy to community engagement, from the role of theory in program development to the key role of design in technology development. The overall picture that emerged from the presentations is of a complex but navigable path toward greater health equity.

CREATING A MOVEMENT FOR CHANGE

"Why do we think digital strategies will make a difference in addressing health disparities?" asked Ivor Horn, medical director of the Center for Diversity and Health Equity and professor of pediatrics at the University of Washington School of Medicine. "There are so many interventions that have been developed over the years, and yet health disparities persist in racial and ethnic minority communities across the country. How is this different from the behavioral interventions that we have done?" she asked.

First, she said, mobile technologies are different than other innovations in health care. As observed in the keynote addresses (see Chapter 2), racial and ethnic minorities have been early adopters of mobile technologies. With smartphones in particular, racial and ethnic minorities have overtaken whites in their use of the technology.

Second, racial and ethnic minorities are leaders in the online community. For example, African Americans spend more than twice as much time per person on Web-hosting sites compared with the average of all consumers. "Racial and ethnic minorities are not just consumers," said Horn, "They are actually producers of information," which translates into an ability to influence the content of the discussion in mainstream media.

Third, racial and ethnic minorities have a clear interest in using digital health. In a recent survey done by Horn and her colleagues of African American parents in an urban clinic, 90 percent said that they want to receive health information online. Other studies have shown that solid majorities of parents in urban pediatric clinics use smartphones as their primary way of getting online, Horn said, explaining, "Not only are they there, not only are they making a difference, but they are really interested in having a health discussion."

Despite the tremendous opportunity to use digital strategies to address health disparities, progress has been slow. One major problem, Horn observed, is that there is a disconnection between where digital strategies are developed and where the needs are. "The motivation for the development of digital strategies is primarily driven by financial gain rather than improving health outcomes. As a result, there is very little motivation to commit to the sometimes lengthy process . . . of developing an evidence base to determine which tools move the needle. Without evidence, providers are not going to adopt them," she explained.

Another barrier to progress is that the effort to reduce health disparities does not present a common enemy against which multiple stakeholders can rally. Action against climate change faces a similar obstacle, Horn noted. People can take many different approaches to address climate change, from driving an electric car to recycling and composting, but the policy framework and infrastructure do not exist to focus and magnify these efforts.

New technologies are driving a shift in communication, said Horn. In health care, providers are trained to communicate with each other. Now, technology is forcing providers to learn how to communicate with patients and with the community in ways they have not done before. She explained:

> To do this, we have to go to the patient and to the community to understand what the need is, because now they are communicating back to us. We have not necessarily been trained to listen. We have been trained to hear, but we do not listen. We hear what we want to hear through our lens of what we are trained to do and to put it into our differential diagnosis, but then we do not hear the relevant thing that we need to hear because we have already moved on while they are still communicating. We need to start figuring out how to make that paradigm shift.

Digital health strategies need to be grounded in the appropriate infrastructure and policies if they are to be effective, Horn said. Also, to be sustainable, these strategies need to be connected to grassroots efforts, organizations, and infrastructure. "Rosa Parks was not just a seamstress who sat down on the bus and decided she did not want to get up," said Horn. "She was part of a strategic grassroots movement connected to a plan to influence policy and make changes."

Digital health strategies present a unique opportunity to address health disparities, but "we need to leverage the trusted leadership of online racial and ethnic minority communities to draw attention to the injustice of health inequities," Horn stated. Doing so would create a call to action and enable people to become learners in the context of a community where leaders already exist.

As an example, Horn described a series of focus groups on technology use done with sickle cell patients who were transitioning out of pediatric care facilities into adult care facilities. When asked how they already were using technology in their day-to-day lives, focus group members said they were, for example, texting their parents to get lists of medications, or using games to distract themselves when they were having a pain crisis. "Whatever you create needs to be hackable," said Horn, "meaning that the patient who has it needs to be able to make it their own." Horn also works with children as young as 2 years old who are creating digital narratives using a tablet. "They are teaching us how to utilize that tool if we listen, if we look, if we pay attention," she said.

In taking on this kind of work, several important questions need to be answered, Horn noted. Where are the communities online? Who are the leaders in those communities? How can the health care community work with those leaders to ensure the information people receive is the right information?

Partnering with racial and ethnic minority developers needs to be paired with outreach to offline organizations and systems, such as churches and community organizations that can push for better access to health care, Horn said. The Affordable Care Act has increased coverage in particular communities, such as the Hispanic community and states that are offering increased coverage. "We need to encourage patients and communities to drive and push for that and fight for that. Without these tangible, sustainable movements for change, we will just be wearing more stylish Google glasses and quantifying ourselves while people continue to prematurely die all around us," she concluded.

THE VALUE OF THEORIES

"Evidence, as important as it is, is not enough," said Misha Pavel, professor of practice jointly appointed between the College of Computer and Information Sciences and the Bouvé College of Health Sciences at Northeastern University. "It is not enough to know that something worked or it did not work. We need to know why, because if we don't, we don't know what to change," he said.

Technology has the potential to create important changes in behavior over the next decade, and, as Pavel said, "Behaviors are killing us." At least 40 percent of premature mortality is the result of people's behaviors. The problem is that behaviors are hard to change. Sexual behaviors, alcohol and drug use, smoking, a sedentary lifestyle, and even sleeping patterns—which are closely related to stress and its negative consequences—are deeply engrained behaviors.

Human behaviors produce health states and biological indicators that can be measured. However, a connection needs to be drawn between what is being measured and what is of concern, Pavel stated. For example, blood pressure is of interest for what it signifies about the health of the cardiovascular system. "We need to have some way of transforming what we measure to what we want to know," said Pavel, "then we can close the loop and intervene in an optimal way."

The proliferation of mobile technologies can help greatly both with the measures of health indicators and with interventions. Indicators that can be measured range all the way from glucose levels to a person's mood. Mobile technologies also can sense the context a person is in and initiate questions or interventions at the appropriate time. For example, they can remind someone to take a medicine or make a measurement when that person is in the right circumstance.

However, the optimal use of technologies requires having a good theory about why and where they work. A good theory "is going to not only drive your design, but also the questions that you ask," said Pavel.

Even when a theory is wrong, demonstrating that it is wrong can result in progress.

Mobile technologies can be used to do much more than has been done to date, Pavel observed. For example, he described a randomized controlled trial on the use of mobile technologies to change people's weight. One group got a traditional weight control intervention, while another group received an intervention that used mobile technologies. "What we do is build these two process models to characterize outreach performance. Once you have a model, then you can develop the most optimal intervention that maintains the weight," he explained.

A major conclusion was that the use of mobile technologies worked for some people and not for others. The challenge thus has evolved from understanding the behavior of groups to modeling the behaviors of individuals to be able to predict which individuals will benefit from an intervention. Pavel explained, "What we need to do is model [the behavior of] individuals and be able to predict what they will do."

Older people can pose unique problems, Pavel noted in response to a question, because many of them "approach technology with suspicion." For example, one of older patients' highest concerns is cognitive decline. In response, "We use games and cognitive games that enable them to practice various cognitive skills," he noted. Also, using Skype, older patients can find each other and build communities, adding "We would have never been able to anticipate that."

In response to another comment, Pavel pointed to the difficulty of keeping up with technology. A study done of a technology, like personal digital assistants, can be obsolete by the time the study is published because the technology is no longer being used. At the same time, mobile technology provides very rapid access to information and data. "We can collect data in a way we have never been able to do before. As a result, we are beginning to think about randomized controlled trials and evidence gathering as a much more dynamic process. . . . But there is also always going to be a bit of a gap," he noted.

A fundamental need, Pavel concluded, is for a vision of what health care will look like in 20 years. Then steps can be taken to help the system evolve toward that vision. Developing the basic principles that will drive progress entails making difficult social and economic decisions, but "we have to face it," he concluded.

A HEALTH LITERACY PERSPECTIVE ON HEALTH DISPARITIES

"How do you engage providers and patients in digital strategies to promote health equity and reduce disparities?" asked Ruth Parker, professor of medicine, pediatrics, and public health at the Emory University School of

Medicine. The research on this question is nascent, Parker noted, and many questions need to be answered, including the following:

- Which digital strategies would do this?
- What are patient-centered, health-literate digital strategies?
- What is known about the value of strategies, in terms of both quality and cost, as the affordability of health care delivery is addressed?
- How do trust, civility, and social impact—for example, the effects of digital technologies on the environment—come into play?

Parker focused mostly on issues of health literacy during her talk, since, as the Institute of Medicine has observed, "Efforts to improve quality, to reduce costs, and to reduce disparities cannot proceed without simultaneous improvements in health literacy" (IOM, 2004, p. xiv). In an effort to define health literacy, a group of authors in the discussion paper *Ten Attributes of Health Literate Health Care Organizations* identified the following qualities (Brach et al., 2012):

1. Has leadership that makes health literacy integral to its mission, structure, and operations.
2. Integrates health literacy into planning, evaluation measures, patient safety, and quality improvement.
3. Prepares the workforce to be health literate and monitors progress.
4. Includes populations served in the design, implementation, and evaluation of health information and services.
5. Meets the needs of populations with a range of health literacy skills while avoiding stigmatization.
6. Uses health literacy strategies in interpersonal communications, and confirms understanding at all points of contact.
7. Provides easy access to health information and services and navigation assistance.
8. Designs and distributes print, audiovisual, and social media content that is easy to understand and act on.
9. Addresses health literacy in high-risk situations, including care transitions and communications about medicines.
10. Communicates clearly what health plans cover and what individuals will have to pay for services.

Many of these attributes have direct parallels with the health literacy of individuals. As an example, Parker cited the final attribute on coverage and cost. "A lot of the transformation of health care organizations will come with cost transparency," she said, because people do not want to waste money.

The main lesson that Parker drew from this list is that patients are the real experts. As one of Parker's patients once told her, "I know what I know. I also know more than I think I do." Therefore, to work effectively with patients, the health care system will need to partner with them, Parker explained. Health care systems also need to find ways to engage patients more effectively, she said later in response to a question. "I have never heard anybody say, 'I get to go to the doctor today.' It's 'I have to go.' Anything we can do to try to make it engaging, to try to make it more fun, that is a good thing," she said.

She described several projects in which partnerships and engagement led to important advances. During the surge of H1N1 cases in the United States, she and her colleagues worked with the Centers for Disease Control and Prevention to develop an online self-triaging flu website. With input from experts and from interviews with potential users, the developers put together a list of questions that would help someone know whether to go to an emergency room or stay home and treat their aches and fever. "Everybody on my team got the flu, by the way, [but] I feel that you really do have to work with the target population to figure out what is going on," she explained. These conversations require learning to listen. Listening to people "is the hardest part of communication," Parker said, "because we do not always hear what we want to hear."

Another example was text4baby, in which the major mobile carriers in the United States waived the fees for text messages sent to pregnant women and mothers with babies in the first year of life. About 650,000 women signed up to use the system, which is still ongoing. To develop the messages, Parker and her colleagues went into the field and tested the messages with potential users. For example, the original message, "The flu can be dangerous for pregnant women & their babies. Talk to your doctor about seasonal flu & H1N1 flu shots," was changed on the basis of this input to "If you get the flu while you are pregnant, you and your baby can get very sick. Ask your doc if you need a flu shot." Besides changing the message from passive to active voice, the new message provided a more specific action step by asking about getting a flu shot. "We tested all these early messages to get input from the ground before they were launched," said Parker.

Evaluations of the text4baby project have found that text messaging is more common among the high-risk population than among other populations (Gazmararian et al., 2012, 2014; Poorman et al., 2014). In addition, successful enrollment was more likely with higher health literacy.

However, these evaluations also identified several major issues that need to be addressed, including a lack of good theories of behavior change, small sample sizes, high drop-off rates, missing control groups, reliance on self-reports, and a failure to tie outcomes to content. Future research, said Parker, needs to look at such issues as navigating mHealth initiatives despite lower health literacy, the use of prepaid phone cards, the delivery of supplemental information (such as videos, icons, or verbal narratives), better enrollment strategies, the effect on behaviors, and the relative effect of the program at different literacy levels.

Parker also discussed a study of Internet and mobile phone use among older Americans. In a study of about 430 subjects drawn from an academic medical center and four community primary care clinics, a significantly larger fraction of those patients with adequate health literacy had Internet access in their home compared to those with limited health literacy. The same is true for access to the Internet anywhere other than the home. These findings provide many opportunities for continued exploration, Parker noted.

Summing up, Parker pointed to several new directions for research and interventions that could help reduce health disparities. Both high-tech and low-tech solutions need to be evaluated, she said. Patient input and engagement need to be maximized to reflect patients' needs, she added, while more practical metrics of technology use and its impact are developed. Health care providers also need to be educated about patient-centered, health-literate digital strategies, she emphasized, with identification of best practices and the competencies that providers should have. "I have never found a health officer or a medical student who regularly advises patients on where to go for good evidence-based and useful information on the Internet or on their phone," she said.

During the discussion session, Parker pointed briefly to some of the privacy issues associated with digital technologies. For example, her elderly patients often tell her that they would like to send and receive photographs of their medications to know what they should be taking. But health systems are concerned that doing so will raise privacy concerns. Photographing medications and taking pictures of clinical wounds or conditions such as wounds or rashes is "a hot zone for action," she said, "because patients like it and it is user friendly. But systems do not know what to do with that."

She concluded by quoting Kelly Johnson's advice to "keep it simple, stupid." "This is still the hallmark of great design," she said. "Simplicity should be the key goal."

DESIGNING SYSTEMS FOR HEALTH LITERACY AND EQUITY

When the World Wide Web first became widely available in the 1990s, Cameron Norman, principal of CENSE Research + Design and an adjunct professor in the Dalla Lana School of Public Health at the University of Toronto, began working on eHealth literacy, which he defined as "the ability to seek, find, understand, and appraise health information from electronic sources and apply the knowledge gained to addressing or solving a health problem" (Norman and Skinner, 2006, p. e9). But this was early in the history of the Web, he added. Since then, his views have evolved. In a 2011 paper, he wrote:

> Just as the field of eHealth is dynamic and evolving, so too is the context where eHealth literacy is applied and understood. The original [model] of eHealth literacy and the scale used to assess it were developed at a time when the first generation of Web tools gained prominence before the rise of social media. The rapid shifts in the informational landscape created by Web 2.0 tools and environments suggests it might be time to revisit the concept of eHealth literacy and consider what a second release might look like. (Norman, 2011, p. e125)

The Web originally was designed to communicate information to the world. In the health context, the idea was that framing and delivering information the right way would get people to change their behavior. But technologies and platforms such as mobile computing, interactive video, Facebook, and Twitter have changed the Web, Norman said. "Now we realize that it is much more about being able to create part of the conversation and lead the conversation." Many interesting conversations happening today are not being led by experts but by members of the public. The one-way push of information remains part of the picture, but it is just a small part of a much more complicated world.

In an earlier era, communicating was about knowing an audience and addressing it directly. The problem with that view is that addressing an audience requires accepting at the outset the basic premises that unite the audience. "Artists do not address themselves to audiences," Norman said, citing the work of the anthropologist Edmund Snow Carpenter. "They create audiences. The artist talks to himself out loud. If what he has to say is significant, others hear and are affected," he explained.

In the context of health disparities, Norman said that digital media now provide the ability for people to "take ownership of the issues and say, 'If others are not going to do it for us, we will do it for ourselves. We will create our own audiences.'" This is a powerful possibility, said Norman, but it also presents challenges.

First, the volume of content that these technologies can provide is overwhelming. "Does anybody in the room here think that they do not have enough e-mail?" he asked. And e-mail is just one channel. Text messages, Facebook posts, tweets, and other electronic intrusions all compete for one's time.

Second, the systems created around information technologies frame the context of information. Norman quoted the historian of technology Melvin

Kranzberg, who established as his first law of technology that "technology is neither good nor bad; nor is it neutral" (Kranzberg, 1995, p. 5). People are expected to make complex health decisions using sophisticated information that is coming at them at light speed. As people are overwhelmed by the amount and complexity of information they receive, they can be expected to question some of the systems enabled by digital technologies. People need to think about what they are gaining and what they are giving up through their use of technology, Norman observed. "What are we hiring this technology to do?" he asked.

The systems created around technologies also have distinct drawbacks. An example is the ad content and other distractions, such as click bait, transmitted with electronic information to support those communications. Norman explained that "your life is time. The more time you are spending on this, [the more] it is part of your life. But is that the life you want?"

Finally, technology is inserting itself into parts of people's lives that were once technology free, "like walking a dog, or walking across the street with a friend, or spending time with your friends or loved ones, or having lunch, or going on a trip and visiting the sites, or exercising," he noted. New technologies can lock people into systems, Norman stated, and people can no longer think about systemic structures when they are locked into those systems. Health disparities originate in systemic structures and patterns of behaviors, said Norman. These structures include how workplaces, communities, and social systems are set up. Technology has the potential to change these structures and patterns of behavior, he said, "but only if we are thinking about it in those terms."

The only way to change systemic problems is to think and act systemically, Norman explained. That requires individuals making individual choices collectively in collaboration with one another. "We need to be thinking about what are individuals doing, but we cannot do that divorced from the idea of what happens within the networks in which people interact," he noted. What is important is to pay attention to what is adding value, Norman said. People may use a technology in a way that was not planned but that nevertheless adds value to their lives. Also, technologies need to fit into the fabric of everyday life and not be simply an add-on if their use is to be sustainable.

Systemic change also involves the concept of design, said Norman, which he views as a way of creating new things. As Nobel laureate Herbert Simon once observed, "A designer is anyone who devises a course of action that seeks to change current situations into preferred ones" (Simon, 1981, p. 129). Technologies can be designed for the collective well-being, or they can continue to focus people on events. "We need to be clear about our intentions," said Norman, because design is about "making intent come alive."

He closed with an observation that is attributed to Paul Batalden, Professor Emeritus of the Geisel School of Medicine at Dartmouth: "Every system is perfectly designed to get the results it gets." To change the system, he said, "We have to listen, and then we have to lead."

4

Examples of Engaging Racial/Ethnic Minority Communities in Digital Health Strategies

> **Important Points Highlighted by the Speakers**
> - Culturally appropriate interventions delivered through online technologies can meet the information needs of racial and ethnic minority communities. (Ginossar)
> - Challenges include the lack of continuous funding, the fact that local heroes move, and continually changing models and technology. (Ginossar)
> - Community-based participatory research can be a way of connecting technology and community so long as the community is integral to the process. (Baumeister, Ginossar, Loveluck)

Two presentations at the workshop looked in more detail at specific examples of successful efforts to engage racial and ethnic minority communities in digital health strategies. One considered the use of technologies in a Latina immigrant community in New Mexico; the other focused on men who have sex with men (MSM) in the Detroit metropolitan area. Though the targeted populations were quite different, both demonstrated how technology-based interventions can reach communities in ways that more traditional interventions cannot.

REDUCING DIGITAL AND HEALTH INEQUITIES IN LATINA IMMIGRANT COMMUNITIES

Tamar Ginossar, who teaches courses in health communication at the University of New Mexico, offered a specific example of how partnerships between universities and local communities can reduce health disparities. She works with a community group called *La Comunidad Habla*, Spanish for "the community speaks." The goal of the partnership is to reduce disparities in a Latina immigrant community, but the same model can be applied to similar collaborations in many different community settings, Ginossar said.

New Mexico is a majority minority state, with Latinos comprising 47 percent of the population, followed by non-Hispanic whites and Native Americans. The state has one of the highest poverty rates in the nation, which in turn leads to health disparities. It also has the lowest rate of broadband access at home.

La Comunidad Habla works predominantly in Southeast Albuquerque, which is close to the University of New Mexico. Known as the international district in recognition of its diversity, it is the most ethnically diverse area in the state, in part because of its central location and relatively affordable housing. Up to 80 percent of the properties are rentals, "which makes building social capital difficult," said Ginossar, "because people do not own their homes, and they move in and out of the area."

Despite increases in online access, the digital divide persists, she continued. Latinos in particular are digitally marginalized in access to information technologies, in having a lower representation in the information technology workforce, and in their lack of culturally relevant content on the Web. This digital divide has marginalizing social and economic effects. "To make informed decision making, we need access to credible information," Ginossar said, adding, "We know from the general population that people with access to health information online report much better health outcomes. Whom are we leaving out?"

Providing online access to digitally marginalized communities is necessary but not sufficient to bridge the digital divide, she said. Culturally appropriate interventions are needed as well to meet the information needs of these communities, said Ginossar, and these interventions need to provide support and culturally appropriate, low-literacy-level content.

Created in 2002 as a community outreach project of the Young Children's Health Center, a University of New Mexico pediatric clinic, *La Comunidad Habla* was founded as a community digital media group to provide women with technological and health advocacy leadership in the community (Ginossar and Nelson, 2010a,b). It began with evening computer classes in Spanish for women, with child care provided, "which is a crucial component," Ginossar emphasized. The project provided opportunities for community members to access health information and technology, in part through a bilingual online health care resource directory (http://www.mycommunitynm.org). With relatively few financial resources, it reached and trained more than 1,000 community members and providers.

When Ginossar began working with the group, she was very interested in how people were using the Internet for health information seeking. She found that community members were particularly interested in the behavioral health of children. "A lot of parents have questions about the development and behavior of children in all communities. There is still a lot of stigma attached to it and not enough services to access," she explained. A literature review revealed that most children who need evaluation and treatment for behavioral health and developmental disorders do not receive it. Children are typically diagnosed after they enter school, but interventions are often most effective in younger children. "We are missing the crucial years of early intervention," Ginossar said.

The scientific literature also showed that the less stigma parents feel about accessing mental health care for their children and the more knowledge they have about early childhood development and behavior, the more likely they are to access services. To reduce stigma and build knowledge, Ginossar and her colleagues created a collaboration with mental health experts that had two objectives: first, to examine low-income Latina community members' information needs and information sources regarding early childhood behavior and development; second, to develop educational outreach to community members and key stakeholders. Drawing on the results of focus groups conducted both in English and in Spanish, the collaboration created educational materials, including an illustrated story, or *historieta*, that combined education and entertainment.

Ginossar ended by listing some of the future research goals for the collaboration. One is to create a larger intervention to meet parental information needs and decrease the digital divide. This larger intervention could be systematically examined—for example, Ginossar said that she was particularly interested in the differences and similarities between digital and print media, because the community organizations were using both.

The collaboration wants to build additional collaborations with health care providers in the community. It also wants to work with day care centers in the community to reach parents and caretakers. "Day care in this community can be a great place to have interventions, and they are very interested in that because of their needs for accreditation," Ginossaur added.

Challenges include the lack of continuous funding, the fact that local heroes move, and continually changing models and technology. Also, community leaders continue to face various barriers, including a lack of broadband access at home.

Tensions can arise between the different requirements of community organizations and academia, Ginossar acknowledged. A lot of what goes on in academia is not relevant to communities or can take a long time to explain. Community-based participatory research involves two cultures coming together, which requires communication about expectations. For example, academics often move from project to project, which is inconsistent with the cultures of communities. But for academics to avoid what has been called "helicopter research," they need the policy and institutional support to remain involved with communities even after the funding is gone. Ginossar said that she has been fortunate to work for an institution that appreciates community-based participatory research and the time it takes.

Finally, Ginossar laid out a potential model for community–academic collaborations:

- Identify content area with the community.
- Review the literature to support the need.
- Cocreate research questions with the community.
- Build on community models.
- Create multidisciplinary collaborations with health care providers and additional stakeholders.
- Identify funding sources.
- Write grant proposals.
- Write additional grant proposals.
- Hope that your community partners can wait.

A TAILORED WEB-BASED INTERVENTION FOR YOUNG MSM IN SOUTHEAST MICHIGAN

Three-quarters of Michigan's HIV/AIDS cases are in Southeast Michigan, with more than 60 percent of the HIV cases in the Detroit Metro Area accounted for by MSM. Furthermore, six of the nine counties in Southeast Michigan account for the majority of the new cases of chlamydia, gonorrhea, and primary and secondary syphilis. Jimena Loveluck, president/CEO of the HIV/AIDS Resource Center (HARC), and Jose Bauermeister, associate professor of health behavior and health education and the director of the Center for Sexuality and Health Disparities (SexLab) at the University of Michigan School of Public Health, described the tailored Web-based technology they have developed to attack these problems by encouraging HIV and sexually transmitted infection (STI) testing among young MSM between the ages of 15 and 24 years.

Get Connected (Bauermeister et al., 2015a) is an adaptation of the Project Connect Health Systems Intervention (Dittus et al., 2014) developed for adolescent heterosexual populations. The adaptation acknowledged the need to address structural barriers affecting service efforts aimed toward HIV/STI prevention and care among young men who have sex with men (YMSM), and the importance of using technology to reach this population. The intervention was developed through a community-based participatory research approach and was informed by existing mixed-methods data focused on YMSM in Southeast Michigan.

Loveluck briefly laid out some of the principles on which community-based participatory research (CBPR) is based (Israel et al., 1998). CBPR recognizes the community as a unit of identity, builds on strengths and resources within the community, facilitates collaborative and equitable involvement of all partners in all phases of the research, and integrates knowledge and intervention for mutual benefit of all partners. Speaking as a program director, Loveluck said "We have been involved in everything from designing the intervention and study tools to helping to think about coding of data. We have learned a lot along the process—and not just me as the director of the organization but many staff."

In the case of Get Connected, CBPR focuses on issues of concern to the community by addressing structural vulnerability among YMSM of color. It also enables the community to use data to advocate for change. In addition, the program has given HARC an opportunity to showcase its work on a national and even an international scale. As Loveluck said in response to a question, "We have to hold our academic institutions accountable for sharing the resources and providing some of the capacity building in communities. . . . Academic institutions really want to work with community partners, but that has to be done in an equal manner."

Get Connected has looked at both HIV vulnerability and protective factors. The barriers to accessing HIV services include cost, transportation to services, age-related barriers, beliefs and risk perceptions, the perceived credibility and competence of providers, medical mistrust, the difficulty of navigating services, and discrimination. To overcome these barriers, Get Connected brought together a variety of groups, including the SexLab at the University of Michigan, the Center for Health and Communications Research at the University of Michigan, a community advisory board made up of service providers, and a youth advisory board, which helped tailor the messages used in the program. Another component of the program was "secret shoppers" (Bauermeister et al., 2015b)—two men per site who went through the process of HIV and STI testing to rate or evaluate the sites based on a set of criteria.

These criteria included structural characteristics, such as the hours a clinic was open, whether it was close to public transportation, how long testing would take, and information about insurance and fee scales. The evaluators also considered such questions as whether the site was youth friendly, whether it was LGBTQ (lesbian, gay, bisexual, transgender, queer) inclusive, whether it was sex positive in terms of its counseling and messages, and whether it had a focus on goal setting and diversity. "Nobody has stopped to ask what it is like for a young man to go get tested in these settings," Bauermeister pointed out, adding "The trust and respect of the users themselves, and making sure that they are also making decisions, are vital."

Bauermeister described the randomized controlled trial conducted as part of the research project that involved 130 young men in Southeast Michigan who had engaged in sex with a male partner in the past 6 months. One group (the tailored intervention condition) received content developed in the Get Connected project, which is tailored to reflect age, race/ethnicity, sexual identity, history of HIV and STI testing, barriers to testing (such as homelessness, residential instability, or discrimination), sources of support, and personal values. They then received information about the locations of test sites. The comparison condition only received the testing directory. "We thought it would be unethical to not give young men a chance to find out where to get tested," Bauermeister said regarding the inclusion of a testing directory as the comparison group, adding "Even though it makes it harder for us scientifically to find the difference between the arms, from a public health and practice perspective, it is the right thing to do."

Both the tailored site and the test locator conditions had very high satisfaction and acceptability by young men. In addition, 30 days after they had received the intervention, more than 30 percent of the men who received the tailored content had been tested for HIV and/or STIs, "which is huge," according to Bauermeister.[1] The testing identified one previously unknown HIV case and two previously unknown STI cases that were treated. In addition, four HIV-positive participants reported visiting their care providers after participating in the intervention.

A particularly interesting result was a reduction in the number of partners among men in the intervention in the following 30 days. Even among those who did not get tested before the 30-day follow-up, there were clinically meaningful reductions in perceived barriers to testing and fears about getting tested, along with increased urgency to get tested and to talk with partners about testing or delaying sex until each person's status was known.

At the time of the workshop, Get Connected was seeking funding for a demonstration project to expand the program to the Atlanta Metro and the Minneapolis–St. Paul regions. It also was planning to switch from secret shoppers to a Yelp-like review system, collect a greater number of time points postintervention, shift the site more toward videos and interactivity than text, and work to extend it from a mobile-friendly to a mobile-based system.

Bauermeister concluded with several lessons drawn from the experi-

---

[1] In the control group, 28 percent of the men reported getting tested for HIV.

ences with Get Connected. CBPR can be a way of connecting technology and community, but the community needs to be integral to the process. Specific areas of HIV education can be targeted in outreach and testing efforts with providers and clients. And YMSM can be empowered to understand and navigate their testing and counseling sessions.

5

Policy and Technology Perspectives

> **Important Points Highlighted by the Speakers**
> - Social media and mobile technologies generally do not intersect with the large-scale data initiatives being promoted by government policies. (Guillermo, Ziv)
> - Barriers to eHealth adoption include a lack of access to technologies, little interoperability of tools across platforms, the linguistic or cultural competency of tools, limitations caused by disability or technological literacy, patient and physician awareness and incentives, inadequate health literacy, and privacy concerns or distrust. (Guillermo, Raymond)
> - Ways to overcome these barriers include improving the digital literacy of consumers and safety net providers, supporting eHealth tools that feature user-centered design, and supporting technology capacity building for safety net providers. (Guillermo)
> - A registry of commercial products that have viability and reliability would enable patients and providers to find good solutions to their problems. (Guillermo)

Following the presentations of the *La Communidad Habla* and Get Connected programs, the workshop participants turned to the broader policy and technology issues that shape such initiatives. Policy can either support or hinder the use of technology toward achieving and creating health equity, which means that policy actions can be a critical factor in the success of interventions.

TOP-DOWN AND BOTTOM-UP APPROACHES TO POLICY

The integration of health information technology and eHealth is being prompted in part by federal policy, observed Tessie Guillermo, president and CEO of ZeroDivide, which is a mission-driven consulting organization that helps communities transform themselves through the adoption and integration of technology. Health Insurance Portability and Accountability Act (HIPAA) regulations, the Health Information Technology for Economic and Clinical Health (HITECH) Act, incentives for meaningful use of electronic health record (EHR) technologies, and revision of the *International Statistical Classification of Diseases and Related Health Problems* (ICD) all have helped drive the digitization of health care.

Even apart from these policies, the health care industry has been rapidly changing. One new emphasis, as the industry moves away from a fee-for-service model toward a fee-for-value world, is population health management, noted Guillermo. In one formulation of that transition, information technology is at the core of population health management, with data driving a virtuous loop of continuous improvement. But a better way to view this transition is by placing the patient in the center of an integrated health care ecosystem, with technology feeding into the system, said Guillermo. In either formulation, information "is a constant."

Today, the pieces of the health ecosystem are not well connected, Guillermo pointed out. Very few community health centers or primary care medical homes have adopted a working EHR, and most will not achieve meaningful use anytime soon. To navigate the system to achieve good outcomes, reduce costs, and improve care management, patients and health care providers have to navigate around processes that today stand outside an integrated system.

Many of these processes involve technology. Social media promote services to new consumers, enable the sharing of stories, and help build communities. Mobile technologies also can promote services along with extending care and providing customer service. Consumers want to take advantage of these technologies, as surveys have repeatedly documented. The problem, said Guillermo, is that these technologies generally do not intersect with the large-scale data initiatives being promoted by policies. The result is likely to be a "long, expensive, difficult, and complex" process of building capacity and managing change to combine the two separate approaches, she explained.

ZeroDivide has been doing research in recent years on the barriers to greater use of eHealth approaches by low-income, immigrant, non-

English-speaking, disabled, rural, and other underserved populations. As part of this research, it has categorized eHealth tools into three categories of decreasing complexity: messaging tools, disease management tools, and tethered personal health records (PHRs) and patient portals.

The evidence shows that messaging and disease management applications are effective in reaching underserved patients and improving their engagement, Guillermo observed. However, these solutions have yet to be brought to commercial scale by large health systems and insurers. Also, applications tend not to be tied to existing hospital and health system records, which presents challenges. Instead, they have been implemented primarily via pilot programs run by departments of health and academic medical centers. As a result, Guillermo said, "Things that work are not getting fast enough into the hands of people that can use them."

PHRs and patient portals hold significant potential to engage and empower patients, Guillermo said. However, they are generally tied to successful electronic medical record systems, which mean that safety net providers are less likely to offer them. Also, they generally have poor usability and design when compared with Web 2.0 tools and mobile apps. Even within integrated health systems, there are significant demographic disparities in their adoption. "All of these problems are things that we have to address . . . on an industry-wide and a population-wide health scale," she added.

Guillermo cited a number of other barriers to eHealth adoption, including a lack of access to technologies, little interoperability of tools across platforms, the linguistic or cultural competency of tools, limitations caused by disability or technological literacy, patient and physician awareness and incentives, inadequate health literacy, and privacy concerns or distrust. She also pointed to the results of focus group research with racial and ethnic minority women, ages 30 to 64, who were making health decisions in their households and were themselves at risk for a chronic disease. They generally have access to the Internet, "Maybe not the highest speed or most affordable, but they have it," she explained. But they are discouraged by what they see, she said, adding "It doesn't reflect them. They want personalized, culturally competent technology solutions."

In response to a question about privacy concerns, Guillermo pointed in particular to the need for a balance between the fear of data being used for the wrong purpose and the use of data for health equity objectives. Everyone in the health care ecosystem has a responsibility for maintaining the confidentiality of data, she said. Also, technologies can help inform patients about how their data will be used so they can have more control over that use. In contrast, if data are written on paper, "it could just be left on the table," Guillermo noted. Education around privacy, confidentiality, and the regulation of data uses is as important as the development of the tools, she said. "The privacy and security barrier is a major obstacle to get past for certain segments of the population. We need to acknowledge the importance of protecting information and communicate" the security steps being taken, she said.

The focus groups resulted in a set of recommendations that Guillermo cited. One is to improve the digital literacy of both consumers and safety net providers, who are interacting with patients around the use of these tools. Another is to support eHealth tools that feature user-centered design. A third is to support technology capacity building for safety net providers. Today, community health centers are being supported to adopt electronic medical records. However, they are not receiving much support for the testing and use of consumer-facing tools or the other infrastructure tools that support operational processes within their clinics.

Policy approaches can be both top-down and bottom-up, Guillermo noted in closing. Top-down federally instigated policies include meaningful use requirements, innovation grants and funds for eHealth pilots, and a central database or registry of approved education resources and apps. For example, a registry of commercial products that have viability and reliability would enable patients and providers to find good solutions to their problems.

Bottom-up community programs also are important, said Guillermo. These include community-led marketing and awareness campaigns, forums to bring patients and developers together, and community eHealth pilots. Communities and academic institutions could form partnerships to develop these approaches, where funding, intellectual property, and revenue streams are shared.

Increasingly, "There is an attentiveness to the need to bring providers, patients, investors, and innovators together to begin to do deep dives into solving some of these barriers," said Guillermo, adding,

> People have to be open to that, to not stay in their enclaves, where we are comfortable.... The people in this room, you all know that. You are a big part of the solution. I would hope that, because of forums like this, there will be opportunities for more of this to happen in an accelerated way.

THE POLICY PERSPECTIVE FROM AN INTEGRATED HEALTH CARE DELIVERY SYSTEM

Kaiser Permanente has "a lot at stake with regards to eHealth equity," said Brian Raymond, senior health policy consultant at the Kaiser Permanente Institute for Health Policy. Kaiser Permanente operates in seven regions, serving eight states and the District of Columbia, and has more than 10 million members. The intersection of health information technology, health care delivery, and the communities, individuals, and families that the system serves are directly linked to eHealth equity.

Kaiser Permanente has made a very large investment in health information technology. Its EHR system, known as HealthConnect, is deployed in all of its facilities across the nation and is the largest health information technology system in use today in the United States. The system integrates appointments, registration, billing, and back office health care functions; supports inpatient care, outpatient care, and ancillary services; and includes a data repository and patient portal. The system provides patients with secure e-mail to their providers, online access to test results, online appointment scheduling, prescription refills, and video appointments with primary care providers. Today, one-third of Kaiser Permanente's primary care visits are conducted by e-mail, and 27 percent of the HealthConnect transactions were conducted via mobile devices. HealthConnect is "transforming care for our members," said Raymond.

These changes are producing quality improvements in care, explained Raymond. Kaiser Permanente's care ratings for chronic conditions and cancer prevention have risen from the middle of the pack to above the 90th percentile since HealthConnect was implemented. All seven of Kaiser Permanente's Medicare plans are among the top 10 plans, as determined by the National Committee for Quality Assurance, and the Southern California plan has been the top-rated plan for the past 3 years.[1]

Despite these quality improvements, "health disparities persist among Kaiser Permanente members," Raymond observed. He showed a series of charts documenting differences in the occurrence of obesity, asthma, diabetes, and hypertension in the San Francisco Bay Area, with areas of poor health corresponding largely with low-income communities and communities of color. "That is a major concern for us," he said.

To ensure the benefits of health information technologies accrue to all its members, not just those with access to technologies and the resources and skills to use them, Kaiser Permanente researchers have been studying potential disparities in the use of HealthConnect by its members. For example, Zhou et al. (2010) found that secure e-mail use by patients was associated with a 2.0 to 6.5 percent improvement in performance on measures of the Healthcare Effectiveness Data and Information Set, such as glycemic (HbA1c), cholesterol, and blood pressure screening and control measures. This finding highlights outcome disparities between users and nonusers of secure e-mail, Raymond observed.

Research also has demonstrated that Kaiser Permanente members who are registered for access to their personal health records are more likely to

---

[1] Kaiser Permanente, unlike other health systems, is not based on a fee-for-service model; this may contribute to their innovations and investments to reduce disparities.

be non-Hispanic whites than the nonusers of the system. Similarly, African Americans and Latinos in northern California were more likely than non-Hispanic whites to request a password for the patient portal but never log on. A study in Georgia found that Kaiser Permanente members with a postgraduate education more frequently registered for access to the patient portal than adults with a high school education or less. "Together, these findings document to us that there are potential eHealth disparities among our membership," said Raymond, adding "This is a concern that we need to keep on our radar and track and address."

To reduce these disparities, Kaiser Permanente has identified and implemented actionable strategies to ensure that health information technology addresses the needs of at-risk and traditionally underserved populations. One approach has been to segment the at-risk population into three groups: "haves" who currently have information technology access and want to use it for their health, "wants" who want access to eHealth and could have it if they receive appropriate assistance, and "don't wants" who do not want access to eHealth. For the "haves," the strategy is to focus on content and functionality—for example, making sure that the patient portal has information that is accessible, useful, and relevant to that population. Marketing is also important for these individuals, in that they may not be aware that a patient portal exists or that it may have content that is valuable to them.

For the "wants," the strategy is to focus on increasing technology access and skill development, such as through a broadband or computer access program in an underserved area or a computer literacy program. A secondary strategy for this segment is to offer alternatives to technology by providing high-quality care and services through low-technology communication channels.

For the "don't wants," high-quality alternatives to technology also are needed, Raymond observed, including traditional in-person visits, phone calls, and print material. Also for this segment, marketing could raise their awareness of the potential value of eHealth to them. "Maybe if it is not to them, it is for a caregiver," Raymond said. "Maybe they are not interested themselves, but they have a proxy who would be interested in using the system on their behalf," he added.

Kaiser Permanente does not have all the answers to eHealth equity, but it has "skin in the game," said Raymond. "We recognize that we have a role to continue playing in terms of advancing research and better understanding both the benefits of our health information technology system and the potential risk that it poses."

OBSERVATIONS FROM A TECHNOLOGY DEVELOPER

At the technology conferences he attends, presenters sometimes ask for a show of hands to determine how many people use iPhones, Android phones, or Windows phones, noted Noam Ziv, the founder and CEO of Kesembe, Inc. But if someone asked an audience to hold up their hands if they had ever been sick, every hand would be raised. For that reason, the integration of technology into health care is obviously of interest to technology developers.

Ziv offered several observations about technology and health based on his experiences and what he had heard at the workshop. He began by noting that communication is the most prevalent utility in the world. Even in places where there is no electricity, people still use cell phones, adding that "They have solar chargers. They find ways to share cell phones. It is absolutely amazing."

Technology developers tend to think in terms of scalability. If adding another person to a service requires hiring a person to support that service, "it is not going to scale," said Ziv. Today, eHealth applications tend to require a high level of expertise to use, which requires extensive support. The way to reach large populations and reduce costs is to have fewer people serving larger populations. This requires making technologies more accessible and usable at all education levels. "Literacy can be improved, but also things can be simplified," he said. iPads, for example, do not ship with manuals because they are designed to work as soon as they are turned on.

The cost of technologies has been declining, Ziv pointed out, but the cost of connectivity, especially in the United States, has not. The United States is not a low-cost wireless or Internet provider; nor is it the world's leader in speed or coverage. The environment that keeps connectivity costs high could be changed, Ziv noted, but doing so requires changing regulations. For example, regulations about what people can store on their phones increases complexity and costs. New policies also could help in places where connectivity is slow or nonexistent.

Much more of health care can move online, Ziv noted. He explained:

> Think about what the banks have done for us. It used to be that whenever you wanted a transaction, you would go to the bank. There will be a teller, one-to-one. You would stand in line. You would tell them, "I would like to deposit a check, . . . what is the balance of my account?"

Today, people get their banking information online, deposit checks electronically, and use automated teller machines for cash. They go to their banks only on rare occasions.

"We have to create similar analogies for health care systems," said Ziv.

"We need to be able to deposit our health data electronically. We need to be able to interact with our health information or health systems when and where and how it is convenient to us. To do that, we need to be able to automate more of these processes," he added.

Technologies also can benefit health care providers by helping them make medical recommendations and eliminating wrong answers. Developing such applications poses challenging and complex problems, Ziv acknowledged, pointing to regulatory hurdles that essentially say, "you can't make a medical recommendation as a machine" without going through a daunting approval process. But regulations could be changed to enable such advances. Also, as Ziv pointed out, not everything can be regulated. People need to learn about the perils as well as the promises of technology.

Finally, companies are interested in health technologies because of the business opportunities they provide. For example, companies are offering cloud-based Web services partly because of the demand for those services but also to build markets for their products. Ziv also mentioned the Qualcomm Tricorder XPrize, which is a $10 million global competition to stimulate innovation and integration of precision diagnostic technologies.[2] The device has to be operable by a patient, not a trained physician, which will improve both usability and health literacy.

---

[2] More information is available at http://tricorder.xprize.org (accessed May 18, 2016).

6

Synthesis of Workshop Messages

In the final session of the workshop, two respondents reflected on the main messages that they heard in the presentations and discussions over the course of the day. Hayley Thompson is associate professor in the department of oncology at the Wayne State School of Medicine and has done research on the use of digital technologies with cancer patients. Andre Blackman is a consultant with the firm Pulse + Signal and co-founder of the FastForward Health Film Festival. Several roundtable members also participated in the conversation, resulting in a wide-ranging summary and extension of the day's discussions.

GENERATING EVIDENCE OF EFFECTIVENESS

Interventions need evidence that demonstrates their effectiveness, said Thompson. Yet the time from "discovery to dissemination" can be an issue for interventions. Creating an evidence-based program requires getting support for the program, implementing it, gathering and analyzing data, demonstrating efficacy, and moving toward dissemination. The length of this process can be daunting for academic researchers, who need to produce results to advance in their careers. Yet academic researchers need to be involved in the process of generating evidence because of the expertise, theory, and methods that they can contribute, Thompson said. Institutions therefore may need to do more to support researchers who want to pursue this work.

One way to involve institutions is to do more education about community-based participatory research. For this research to succeed, said

Thompson, institutional review boards, reviewers, and other parts of the research ecosystem need to know more about the methods, practices, and processes of this research.

At the same time, research could be sped up through innovative approaches. Traditional randomized controlled trials are not always necessary to demonstrate efficacy, Thompson observed. Methods like pragmatic trials, comprehensive dynamic trials, or rapid learning cycles can produce valuable evidence and move the field forward.

PRIVACY AND SUSTAINABILITY

Blackman began by emphasizing the intersection of policy and privacy, which came up periodically during the workshop. eHealth applications generate data that are both medically and commercially valuable. Companies such as Apple are paying attention to how data from digital health applications are shared. But patients need to have control over the sharing of information, he said.

He also pointed toward the importance of sustainability. People's lives are so full, change is so rapid, and people are exposed to so much information that a short-term campaign cannot be expected to have a lasting effect. Instead, sustainability needs to be integrated into interventions, he said, so that change is built into the context of people's lives. The design of an intervention can be a critical factor in its sustainability, he pointed out, and guides to human-centered design exist and could be used toward this end.

THE IN-PERSON COMPONENT

Technology is a valuable tool, said Blackman, but it cannot replace person-to-person contact, especially in communities likely to experience health disparities. "There is no substitute for getting down and talking to people about how this is going to be useful, why this is important in your lives, why it is important for your family, and getting feedback from them." The two-way exchange of information requires listening and finding out what is important in people's lives. "That is where we can begin to tailor a lot of these initiatives and tools around what is actually important in people's lives," he explained.

Health is something that people tend not to think about when they are feeling fine, but people need to be engaged even when health is not forefront in their minds, said Blackman. Integrating health into the things that are forefront in their mind would be one way to pursue this goal. A single father with three children who is working multiple jobs does not have time to think about eating five fruits and vegetables per day. But if healthy eating could be made part of the issues that concern such a father, progress could be made. Also, the social determinants of health are extremely powerful, Blackman reminded the workshop participants. Thinking about how health interacts with transportation, family issues, or other things that are important in people's lives could improve health while addressing nonhealth issues as well.

Focusing on the social determinants of health emphasizes the importance of multidisciplinary research, Thompson added. She is a psychologist who partners with anthropologists so they can go into people's homes and figure out how technology fits into their lives and can more effectively meet their needs. For this kind of research, a multidisciplinary perspective is critical, she said. The use of technology in health care also requires the use of people throughout a community, such as community health workers and community leaders, she said. This is particularly the case with the most marginalized communities, such as people involved with substance abuse, the criminal justice system, or the foster system.

INVOLVING COMMUNITIES

Thompson returned to the need to fully engage community members and stakeholders in the process of tool development and tool evaluation. Furthermore, communities are not just the people who live in specific neighborhoods. Online communities, thought leaders, and content creators are examples of dispersed communities that can help build a movement for the use of technology to reduce health disparities. A useful guide, she added in response to a question, is critical race theory,[1] especially in its application to public health.

Involving communities means arranging for feedback from community members at all stages of a project, Blackman said, adding "From the jump, we need to make sure that the people who we are looking to serve are a part of it . . . so that we are able to create things that matter." Such feedback can contribute to the rapid development of a program, even if it means that a program fails quickly so developers can pursue other ideas.

Blackman also cited several additional communities that should be involved, such as racial and ethnic minority technology entrepreneurs, educators, and workforce development organizers. "Introduce yourself to these kinds of leaders; let them know what you are about," and then let them help you, he said.

Winston Wong, medical director for Kaiser Permanente Community

---

[1] Critical race theory looks at the relationships among race, racism, and power. It is an activist approach that is based on the assumptions that racism is ordinary and acceptable, white privilege exists, and the belief that the concepts of race and racism are social constructs rather than a biological reality.

Benefit, commented on the need for technology companies to be more accountable to the diversity of American society. These firms can create opportunities for diverse groups to help create and use technologies. In this way, they can address some of the broader determinants of health that help generate disparities. The guiding principle, he said, should be "no technology without me."

SCALABILITY AND ADAPTABILITY

An interesting discussion took place regarding the extent to which an intervention can be scaled up without losing the cultural competency that helped make the original intervention effective. Thompson emphasized the importance of building feedback into an intervention so it can be adapted to new circumstances while it is being scaled up.

Mildred Thompson asked if scalability is always possible: "If I create a community-based program here in the city of Detroit, and I have worked with my community partners and members, and we have some effective outcomes in terms of health—and we have worked closely for years on this initiative—why would I expect that to work in exactly the same way in Chicago?" A better way to think about scalability may be in terms of the methods, ideas, and templates that people elsewhere can use to design their own intervention. In particular, added Toni Villarruel, Dean of the University of Pennsylvania School of Nursing, there may be critical elements that need to be sustained while other elements can be changed. "We, as researchers, have the obligation to help people figure out what we have learned and how that can be used in their community," she said.

INVOLVING PROVIDERS

Finally, Thompson pointed to an obstacle not much discussed at the workshop, which is the willingness of health care providers to accept and adopt technologies. "Some of our research across institutions here in Detroit shows that there is not always uniform acceptance of a new technology" by providers, she said. Providers may see new technologies as taking valuable time to learn and to use, even when they are beneficial to patients. At Kaiser Permanente, the use of technology is "part of the organizational culture, but that is not the case everywhere," she concluded.

References

AHRQ (Agency for Healthcare Research and Quality). 2013. *National Healthcare Disparities Report 2012* No 13-0003: Washington, DC.

Bauermeister, J. A., E. S. Pingel, L. Jadwin-Cakmak, G. W. Harper, K. Horvath, G. Weiss, and P. Dittus. 2015a. Acceptability and preliminary efficacy of a tailored online HIV/STI testing intervention for young men who have sex with men. *AIDS & Behavior* 19(10):1860-1874.

Bauermeister, J. A., E. S. Pingel, L. Jadwin-Cakmak, S. Meanley, D. Alapati, M. Moore, M. Lowther, R. Wade, and G. W. Harper. 2015b. The use of mystery shopping for quality assurance evaluations of HIV/STI testing sites offering services to young gay and bisexual men. *AIDS & Behavior* 19(10):1919-1927.

Brach, C., D. Keller, L. M. Hernandez, C. Baur, R. Parker, B. Dreyer, P. Schyve, A. J. Lemerise, and D. Schillinger. 2012. *Ten attributes of health literate health care organizations.* Discussion paper. Washington, DC: Institute of Medicine.

Cisco. 2015. *Cisco announces intent to acquire OpenDNS.* newsroom.cisco.com (accessed May 18, 2106).

Dittus, P. J., C. J. De Rosa, R. A. Jeffries, A. A. Afifi, W. G. Cumberland, E. Q. Chung, E. Martinez, P. R. Kerndt, and K. A. Ethier. 2014. The Project Connect health systems intervention: Linking sexually experienced youth to sexual and reproductive health care. *Journal of Adolescent Health* 55(4):528-534.

Gazmararian, J. A., B. Yang, L. Elon, M. Graham, and R. Parker. 2012. Successful enrollment in Text4Baby more likely with higher health literacy. *Journal of Health Communication* 17(Suppl. 3):303-311.

Gazmararian, J. A., L. Elon, B. Yang, M. Graham, and R. Parker. 2014. Text4baby program: An opportunity to reach underserved pregnant and postpartum women? *Maternal and Child Health Journal* 18(1):223-232.

Ginossar, T., and S. Nelson. 2010a. La Comunidad Habla: Using Internet community-based information interventions to increase empowerment and access to health care of low income Latino/a immigrants. *Communication Education* 59(3):328-343.

Ginossar, T., and S. Nelson. 2010b. Reducing the health and digital divides: A model for using community-based participatory research approach to E-health interventions in low income Hispanic communities. *Journal of Computer Mediated Communication* 15(4):530-551.

IOM (Institute of Medicine). 2002. *Unequal treatment: Confronting racial and ethnic disparities in health care.* Washington, DC: The National Academies Press.

IOM. 2004. *Health literacy: A prescription to end confusion.* Washington, DC: The National Academies Press.

IOM. 2011. *Digital infrastructure for the Learning Health System: The foundation for continuous improvement in health and health care: Workshop series summary.* Washington, DC: The National Academies Press.

Israel, B. A., A. J. Schulz, E. A. Parker, and A. B. Becker. 1998. Review of community-based research: Assessing partnership approaches to improve public health. *Annual Review of Public Health* 19:173-202.

Kranzberg, M. 1995. Technology and history: "Kranzberg's laws." *Bulletin of Science, Technology, and Society* 15(1):5-13.

Norman, C. 2011. eHealth literacy 2.0: Problems and opportunities with an evolving concept. *Journal of Medical Internet Research* 13(4):e125.

Norman, C. D., and H. A. Skinner. 2006. eHealth literacy: Essential skills for consumer health in a networked world. *Journal of Medical Internet Research* 8(2):e9.

Poorman, G., Elon, R. Parker. 2014. Is health literacy related to health behaviors and cell phone usage patterns among the text4baby target population? *Archives of Public Health* 72(1):13.

Simon, H. A. 1981. *The sciences of the artificial*, 2nd ed. Boston, MA: MIT Press.

Zhou, Y. Y., M. H. Kanter, J. J. Wang, and T. Garrido. 2010. Improved quality at Kaiser Permanente through e-mail between physicians and patients. *Health Affairs (Millwood)* 29(7):1370-1375.

A

Examples of eHealth Solutions Featured at the Workshop

COMMUNITY HEALTH ENGAGEMENT SURVEY SOLUTIONS (CHESS)

Denise Stevens, Matrix Public Health Solutions

Community Health Engagement Survey Solutions (CHESS) is a novel "mHealth" or mobile health strategy for addressing gaps in racial and ethnic health equity developed by Matrix Public Health Solutions in New Haven, Connecticut. CHESS partners with nonprofit youth groups and community improvement organizations to collect data on the neighborhood environment using mobile technology. These data provide a starting point for dialogue and strategic planning to take action on health promotion and disease prevention in the neighborhood.

CHESS's mobile technology tools include surveys and geographic information system (GIS) mapping to systematically assess four health risk factors in a neighborhood: food, physical activity, tobacco, and alcohol. Participants such as a youth "health explorer" team in the Williamsburg neighborhood of Brooklyn, were trained to use a CHESS app on a digital tablet to survey the streets, food stores, restaurants, fitness facilities, and parks, among other features, within a 400-meter walking radius of their school. The work helped the youth to understand how the environments where they live encourage or discourage healthy eating, physical activity, and tobacco use, which in turn influences their behavior and resulting health.

CHESS analyzes and interprets the gathered data through visual maps and quantitative summaries and then, based on that evidence, applies public health expertise to identify potential strategies for intervention and community development to improve access to healthy food and opportunities for physical activity in the neighborhood. For more information, visit http://www.matrixphc.com/chess and watch a video at vimeo.com/104497828.

DOUBLE UP FOOD BUCKS

Liz Kohn, Fair Food Network

Double Up Food Bucks (http://doubleupfoodbucks.org) is a healthy food incentive project of the Fair Food Network, a national nonprofit based in Ann Arbor, Michigan. Launched in 2009, Double Up makes it easier for low-income families in the federal food stamp program—the Supplemental Nutrition Assistance Program (SNAP)—to eat fresh fruits and vegetables while supporting local farmers and economies. When recipients spend SNAP dollars at farmers' markets, they receive up to $20 of matching credit in Double Up Food Bucks that they can use to buy additional Michigan-grown produce. The project has been an innovator in developing new mobile payment processing technology for use at the markets.

Since its initial start in five farmers' markets in Detroit, Double Up has spread to more than 150 sites across Michigan and northern Ohio with the help of funding from George Soros's Open Society Foundations. In 5 years, the project tallied more than 200,000 SNAP/Double Up customer visits at participating sites and more than $5 million of income earned for Michigan farmers and vendors. In 2013, Double Up began expanding into some grocery stores in a partnership with the U.S. Department of Agriculture.

The Double Up model includes a uniform design and brand, centralized administration, and a comprehensive communications strategy, including dynamic social marketing. It depends on strong partnerships with local and statewide organizations and agencies. Evaluation work shows that SNAP customers at farmers' markets report eating more produce and buying fewer unhealthy snacks.

EATFRESH.ORG

Adrienne Markworth, Leah's Pantry

EatFresh.org is a healthy eating resource that offers multilingual information via its website, social media, and mobile technology to low-income Californians who receive food stamp assistance through CalFresh and SNAP. Funded with support from the Aetna Foundation, the website is a project of the Human Services Agency of the City and County of San Francisco, with nutrition and culinary content managed by Leah's Pantry (http://leahspantrysf.org/what-we-do-1). The EatFresh site launched in October

2013 with the goal of encouraging cooking at home with fresh foods and minimally processed, nonperishable ingredients. Content can be viewed in Chinese, English, and Spanish.

The website has more than 400 recipes for tasty and healthy yet affordable dishes as well as a "Discover Foods" section that gives basic information on food ingredients. EatFresh hopes to help users better understand the link between lifestyle or diet choices and prevention of chronic diseases, and to show them that healthy change can happen even though barriers exist. The site also offers healthy lifestyle tips and an "Ask the Dietitian" community forum.

CalFresh, county health departments, food banks, and other agencies around California have integrated EatFresh.org as a nutrition education tool. As of September 2014, nearly 45,000 unique visitors had frequented the EatFresh.org website, 25 percent of them through a smartphone. Users may sign up to receive weekly EatFresh tips via e-mail or text. The project's educational materials are available at http://leahspantrysf.org/eatfresh-toolkit.

FIND MI CARE

Hanna Harp, Greater Detroit Area Health Council

Find MI Care is a free website and mobile application that simplifies the task of finding local, low-cost health care in Michigan. Recognizing a need for patients to receive better coordinated health care treatment close to home, the nonprofit Greater Detroit Area Health Council—a coalition addressing health care quality, access, and cost in Southeast Michigan—created this search tool with a grant from the Robert Wood Johnson Foundation. Visitors to the www.findMIcare.org website can select the health services they are looking for from a menu of options (ranging from primary care and specialty services to medication assistance), and then specify their zip code or region. A list of clinics in the area is generated, with a brief description of each facility and important notes, such as whether it provides care to uninsured individuals. Hospitals, physicians, and community groups can use Find MI Care to help connect Michigan residents to health care resources. The tool can be downloaded as a free smartphone app.

GET CONNECTED

Jose Bauermeister, University of Michigan School of Public Health
Jimena Loveluck, HIV/AIDS Resource Center

Get Connected is a tailored, Web-based health intervention that aims to increase awareness about sexually transmitted illnesses (STIs) among young men who have sex with men (YMSM), and to link them to health clinics that can provide testing for those diseases in a culturally sensitive manner. This work builds upon an existing community-based participatory research project on HIV and STIs at the University of Michigan. Researchers at the university's Center for Health Communications Research and the Center for Sexuality & Health Disparities created the Get Connected website with support from the Centers for Disease Control and Prevention and the National Association of County and City Health Officials.

Get Connected seeks to reach young gay or bisexual men in Southeast Michigan who use e-technologies such as websites and smartphones to meet partners. The Web intervention was developed with input from a youth advisory board, community provider advisors, and local HIV/AIDS organizations. The website provides information on STIs, walks users through the thought process of why they would or would not wish to undergo testing, and uses tailored messaging on values and barriers to try to motivate them to get tested.

Get Connected also offers an STI testing-site search tool that helps users find high-quality, local clinics with the services they need, and the website generates a list of questions, which users can print out or receive by e-mail or text to ask the health provider during their appointment. The researchers have been studying whether Get Connected effectively increases STI testing among the website's users (see http://chcr.umich.edu/project.php?id=1108), and the researchers are expanding their intervention to mobile devices.

LET'S GET HEALTHY! AND 5-2-1-0 KIDS!

Sharon Milberger, Henry Ford LiveWell

Let's Get Healthy! is a healthy living education program developed for overweight children ages 9 to 13 by the Henry Ford Health System's LiveWell division. The 10-week program partners each youngster with a parent to work with a multidisciplinary team that includes a pediatrician, behavioral therapist, registered dietitian, and athletic trainer. This team offers guidance and insight, with a goal of education and behavioral changes rather than weight loss. The dietitian helps each family to build healthy meal plans and realistic lifestyle changes. The team instructors try to convey engaging messages to reshape the way the child thinks about food, nutrition, and exercise.

Participants learn about mindful eating, portion sizes, label reading, fast food and snack choices, quick and healthy meals, smart grocery shopping, and maintaining a food journal. Behavioral modifications are encouraged through setting goals and maintaining and celebrating successes, and through conversations on topics such as staying motivated, stress, and time

APPENDIX A

management. Kids and families also learn fun and affordable ways to exercise and tips on maintaining an active lifestyle.

Let's Get Healthy! recommends the "5-2-1-0" guidelines for daily nutrition and fitness: 5 fruits and vegetables, 2 hours or less of screen time, 1 hour or more of physical activity, and 0 sugar-added beverages. Henry Ford LiveWell has created a fun, interactive game app called "5-2-1-0 Kids!" with messages about eating right and staying active. Families can download the game for free from the Apple and Android app stores. For more information about Let's Get Healthy! visit http://henryfordlivewell.com/body.cfm?id=991&fr=true.

MOBILE DAD

Shawna Lee, University of Michigan School of Social Work

Mobile Dad (mDad) Baby Book is an interactive mobile technology application that enhances the engagement of fathers with their families. Researchers at the University of Michigan created this smartphone app at the request of the U.S. Air Force (USAF) to help military members who are fathers stay involved with their young children while deployed away from home, and to ease the transition when they come back.

Mobile Dad is a cross between a digital baby book and a parent education resource, and fathers can use it independently or with spouses or partners. The app allows users to upload pictures, videos, and audio recordings of their child to track his or her growth. Twice a week, fathers receive brief messages on their iPhone, iPad, or iPod Touch that are tailored to their child's age and developmental milestones. If an infant turns 6 months old, for instance, the parent will receive a notification that the baby can soon start eating solid food. The app can provide more detailed information about that milestone, along with tips on parenting and fun activities to support the child's healthy growth.

The app is tailored for helping fathers balance military and family life, and users can benefit from advice shared by other military dads. mDad was field tested with 200 USAF mothers and fathers. For more information, visit http://chcr.umich.edu/project.php?id=1104.

PLAN PILOT

Tessie Guillermo, ZeroDivide

Plan Pilot is a prototype mobile technology application that draws on health plan datasets to make shopping for health insurance an easier and less confusing experience. It was developed by the San Francisco–based consulting organization ZeroDivide, which seeks to transform underserved communities through technology, including eHealth or electronic health resources tools. The Plan Pilot app is a finalist in the Plan Choice Challenge sponsored by the Robert Wood Johnson Foundation in summer 2014 to spark the development of new apps and tools that allow consumers to compare costs, features, and ratings of health insurance plans and choose the best plan to suit their needs in the new marketplaces created by the Affordable Care Act (ACA). App developers were given access to a set of data on cost-sharing features of plans offered in the health insurance marketplaces in every state and Washington, DC.

ZeroDivide describes Plan Pilot as "a responsive Web application that helps consumers make wise decisions, live healthier lives, and save money on the true total cost of health care." Many Americans who enrolled in health plans through the insurance marketplaces under the ACA have reported dissatisfaction with their choice, and only 60 percent were confident they would be able to pay for a major illness or injury. ZeroDivide's consumer research identified confusion, complexity of choices, and poor customer experiences as the major challenges in making good decisions about buying health insurance. The Plan Pilot app will help users "navigate their health care coverage with personalized recommendations about plan and provider quality as well as savings for prescription drugs."

Y-MVP TEEN FITNESS CHALLENGE

Lori Benson, YMCA of Greater New York

The Y-MVP Teen Fitness Challenge is an 8-week YMCA training program that is innovatively integrated with a digital game to get teenagers engaging in moderate to vigorous physical (MVP) activity every day. The YMCA of Greater New York developed the challenge to incorporate online game design techniques that grab the interest of young people. What started as a pilot program in spring 2013 at the Bedford-Stuyvesant Y in Brooklyn and the Harlem Y in Manhattan is expanding to all YMCA sites across New York City by 2015.

Teens who register for Y-MVP meet once per week in small classes with a trained coach who takes them on a series of fitness "quests" or activities. At the end of each session, participants are assigned a fitness "mission" that they must complete before they meet next. An accompanying interactive digital app and a dynamic badge system tracks, motivates, and rewards the teens' efforts. The youths access the Y-MVP app on a tablet at the gym to record their workouts and monitor their progress toward successfully reaching the activity goals set by their coach. Along the way, they earn and

APPENDIX A

accumulate digital badges that can ultimately be exchanged for incentives such as t-shirts and water bottles. Participants share their accomplishments on social media sites.

Y-MVP is supported by Aetna Foundation, American Express, the Hive Digital Media Learning Fund, and the PepsiCo Foundation. For more details, visit http://www.ymcanyc.org/association/pages/y-mvp or watch a video at www.youtube.com/watch?v=9x7t2k_4Kdo&feature=youtu.be.

B

Workshop Agenda

Digital Health Strategies, Health Disparities, and Health Equity: The Promises and Perils of Technology: A Public Workshop

October 2, 2014
The Margherio Family Conference Center
403 East Canfield Street
Wayne State University
Detroit, MI

Objectives of the Meeting

- To discuss the opportunities to use digital health technologies as a population health strategy to reduce health disparities and promote health equity in the United States.
- To explore how racial and ethnic minority populations/communities in the United States can be engaged in efforts that use digital health strategies to reduce racial and ethnic health disparities.
- To develop effective strategies that engage racial and ethnic minority populations/communities in using digital health strategies to reduce health disparities and promote health equity.
- To explore the different types of digital health technologies used in efforts to reduce health disparities and promote health equity in the United States.
- To highlight examples of digital health strategies designed to reduce health disparities and promote health equity in the United States.

8:00 am	**Welcome and Introduction**
	Toni Villarruel, Ph.D., FAAN, Professor and Margaret Bond Simon Dean of Nursing, University of Pennsylvania School of Nursing
	Gillian Barclay, D.D.S., Dr.P.H., Vice President, Aetna Foundation
	M. Roy Wilson, M.D., M.S., President, Wayne State University
8:30 am	**Keynote: Overarching Views**
	Kimberlydawn Wisdom, M.D., M.S., Senior Vice President of Community Health & Equity and Chief Wellness Officer, Henry Ford Health System, Chair, Gail and Lois Warden Endowment on Multicultural Health
	Wendy Nilsen, Ph.D., Health Scientist Administrator, Office of Behavioral and Social Sciences Research, National Institutes of Health
10:00 am	**Break**
10:15 am	**Panel 1: How do we engage providers and racial and ethnic minority patients in digital strategies with the goal to reduce health disparities and promote health equity?**
	Moderators: Rohit Varma, M.D., M.P.H., University of Southern California, and Winston Wong, M.D., M.S., Kaiser Permanente
	Ivor Horn, M.D., M.P.H., Medical Director of the Center for Diversity and Health Equity and Professor of Pediatrics, University of Washington School of Medicine
	Misha Pavel, Ph.D., Professor of Practice, Northeastern University
	Ruth Parker, M.D., Professor, Emory University
11:30 am	**Discussion with Panel 1**
11:45 am	**Panel 2: How do we engage racial and ethnic minority communities in digital health strategies with the goal to reduce health disparities and promote health equity?**
	Moderator: Caroline McKay, Ph.D., Merck & Co., Inc.
	Cameron Norman, Ph.D., M.A., M.Des., adjunct lecturer, Dalla Lana School of Public Health, University of Toronto
	Tamar Ginossar, Ph.D., Assistant Professor, University of New Mexico

> *Jose Bauermeister, Ph.D., M.P.H., Director, Center for Sexuality & Health Disparities, University of Michigan School of Public Health*
> *Jimena Loveluck, President and Chief Executive Officer, HIV/AIDS Resource Center*

12:45 pm Discussion with Panel 2

1:00 pm Lunch and Technology Speed Dating: Virtual Poster Session
Elliman Building (directly across the street)
- Get Connected!, *Jose Bauermeister, Ph.D., M.P.H., University of Michigan, School of Public Health, and Jimena Loveluck, HIV/AIDS Resource Center*
- EatFresh.org, *Adrienne Markworth, Leah's Pantry*
- PlanPilot, *Tessie Guillermo, ZeroDivide*
- Y-MVP Teen Fitness Challenge, *Lori Benson, YMCA of Greater New York*
- 5-2-1-0 Kids!, *Sharon Milberger, Sc.D., Henry Ford LiveWell*
- Double Up Food Bucks, *Liz Cohn, Fair Food Network*
- Find MI Care, *Hanna Harp, Greater Detroit Area Health Council*
- mDad (Mobile Device Assisted Dad), *Shawna Lee, Ph.D., M.S.W., M.P.P., University of Michigan*
- CHESS, *Denise Stevens, Ph.D., MatrixPHC*

2:45 pm Panel 3: Policy and Technology Perspectives
Moderator: Terri Wright, Ph.D., M.P.H., American Public Health Association
Noam Ziv, Founder, Kesembe Inc.
Brian Raymond, M.P.H., Senior Policy Consultant, Kaiser Permanente Institute for Health Policy
Tessie Guillermo, President and Chief Executive Officer, ZeroDivide

3:45 pm Discussion with Panel 3

4:00 pm Synthesis and Further Discussion Panel
Moderator: Toni Villarruel, Ph.D., FAAN, Professor and Margaret Bond Simon Dean of Nursing, University of Pennsylvania School of Nursing
Andre Blackman, Founder and Chief Executive Officer, Pulse and Signal

> Hayley Thompson, Ph.D., M.S., Associate Professor, Wayne State University School of Medicine

4:45 pm **Concluding Remarks**
> Gillian Barclay, D.D.S., Dr.P.H., Vice President, Aetna Foundation

Roundtable Information

- Project website for the Roundtable on the Promotion of Health Equity and the Elimination of Health Disparities: http://www.nationalacademies.org/hmd/Activities/SelectPops/HealthDisparities.aspx
- The website provides listserv sign-up, information on upcoming meetings, meeting materials such as presentations and webcasts, and roundtable products.
- Project e-mail: healthequityrt@nas.edu

C

Speaker Biographical Sketches

Jose Bauermeister, M.P.H., Ph.D., is the John G. Searle Assistant Professor of Health Behavior and Health Education, and director of the Center for Sexuality & Health Disparities (SexLab) at the School of Public Health. Locally, Dr. Bauermeister has led an academic–community partnership focused on addressing the structural barriers fueling the HIV/sexually transmitted infection (STI) disparities faced by black and Latino young men who have sex with men (YMSM) in the Detroit Metro Area. Dr. Bauermeister is also principal investigator and co-investigator of several projects examining HIV/STI prevention among YMSM, with a focus on how to integrate existing (e.g., condom use) and forthcoming (e.g., Pre-Exposure Prophylaxis; rectal microbicides) prevention technologies into HIV/STI prevention for YMSM. In light of his expertise, he serves as a member of the Behavioral Science Working Group of the Microbicides Trials Network. Dr. Bauermeister is also co-investigator on several projects examining the social and behavioral correlates of young adult well-being, as measured by HIV/AIDS risk, substance use, and psychological well-being. He is co-investigator of the Pediatric HIV/AIDS Cohort Study, one of the largest prospective biomedical studies of perinatally infected adolescents in the United States. Dr. Bauermeister serves on the editorial boards of the *Journal of Youth & Adolescence*, *Archives of Sexual Behavior*, *AIDS and Behavior*, and *Health Education & Behavior*. He is chair of the American Public Health Association's HIV/AIDS Section.

Andre Blackman is a connected agent of change within the health community. He is very interested in the intersection of media, technology, and design as it relates to the sustainable improvement of public health and health care, as well as the stories that result from these new ideas. Through his consulting firm, Pulse + Signal, Andre aims to empower a new generation of thought leaders to do great work through digital branding, effective coaching, and strategic digital public relations/communications. He is passionate about purposefully connecting the organizations and leaders changing the health landscape in our society with the resources to create sustainable change. Andre has been involved in traditional and digital campaigns for the Centers for Disease Control and Prevention and the National Institutes of Health focused on areas such as disease informatics, HIV/AIDS, and diabetes. Andre also serves on the following advisory boards: Mayo Clinic Center for Social Media; SXSW Interactive Conference Advisory Board; Center for Health Media & Policy; National Health Communications, and Marketing and Media Conference. He is the co-founder of the FastForward Health Film Festival—an event dedicated to highlighting the stories of forward thinking in health initiatives around the world.

Tamar Ginossar, Ph.D., teaches courses in health communication, including a class about health, culture, and diversity as part of the B.A./M.D. program at the University of New Mexico. Additional courses include advanced quantitative research methods, intercultural communication, and organizational communication. Dr. Ginossar has held two previous faculty appointments at the Department of Communication in Tel Aviv University and as research faculty with the University of New Mexico School of Medicine. Her research interests focus on health communication and reducing health disparities. She is particularly interested in how communities and individuals are using new communication technologies for information exchange and advocacy. She lived and traveled internationally in the Middle East, Europe, Asia, and Latin America. Her research focuses on health communication and reducing health disparities. More specifically, Dr. Ginossar is interested in how communities and individuals are using new communication technologies for information exchange and advocacy, and in how they seek and share information, and in designing interventions using community-based research approaches to reduce health disparities.

Tessie Guillermo is the president and CEO of ZeroDivide, a consulting organization focusing on technology adoption and innovation to improve health, economic opportunity, and civic engagement of disadvantaged communities. Ms. Guillermo served for 15 years as CEO of the Asian and Pacific Islander American Health Forum, a national health policy/advocacy organization. She was appointed by President Clinton in 1999 as an inaugural member of the President's Commission on Asian Americans and Pacific Islanders. Ms. Guillermo recently completed a 10-year tenure as a member of the board of directors of The California Endowment, serving for 3 years as chairwoman. She serves as an executive member of the Board for Dignity Health, and is a board member of the Nonprofit Finance Fund and the California State University East Bay Education Foundation, where she graduated with a B.A. in economics. She is a graduate of the Gallup Leadership Institute and was a 1997 fellow of the Asian Pacific American Women's Leadership Institute.

Ivor Horn, M.D., M.P.H., is medical director of the Center for Diversity and Health Equity at Seattle Children's Hospital, and professor of pediatrics at the University of Washington School of Medicine. Dr. Horn is a National Institutes of Health–funded researcher in the area of health communication with underrepresented racial and ethnic minority communities using mobile technology innovations. She is principal investigator on a study of a text-message-based health communication intervention to improve asthma outcomes in an urban disadvantaged population. Dr. Horn was also the project director as part of the collaborative team funded by the Agency for Healthcare Research and Quality (AHRQ) to develop technology-enabled tools to facilitate transitions in care for patients with sickle cell anemia at Children's National Health Systems. The project, a collaboration between Children's National Health Systems, Cincinnati Children's Hospital Medical Center, The Lewin Group, the National Institute for Children's Healthcare Quality, and Nemours, was part of AHRQ's Accelerating Change and Transformation in Organizations and Networks (ACTION) Program. On a national level, Dr. Horn is a board member and communication director for the Academic Pediatric Association (the leading professional organization for general academic pediatrician researchers). Dr. Horn has served as first author on two seminal papers about the approach to child health disparities research. Dr. Horn is also a community-based primary care pediatrician with more than a decade of experience providing care and conducting research in communities of color.

Jimena Loveluck is president/CEO of the HIV/AIDS Resource Center (HARC) in Ypsilanti, Michigan. She has a master's degree in social work from Boston College, specializing in community organization and social policy and planning. After completing her M.S.W. in 1990, Ms. Loveluck began working for the Massachusetts Department of Public Health AIDS Bureau, where she conducted HIV counseling and testing services in hospital and clinic settings, and also staffed the Massachusetts AIDS Hotline. Ms. Loveluck left the state level after 2 years to become director of HIV Services at Whittier Street Neighborhood Health Center, a federally qualified health center in Roxbury, Massachusetts. She returned to Michigan in 1999 and became the president/CEO of the HARC in November 2000. She has been involved in community-based participatory research in collaboration with The Center for Sexuality and Health Disparities at the University of Michigan's School of Public Health since 2009.

Wendy Nilsen, Ph.D., is a health scientist administrator at the National Institutes of Health (NIH) Office of Behavioral and Social Sciences Research and the program director for the Smart and Connected Health program at the National Science Foundation (NSF). Dr. Nilsen's scientific focus is on the science of human behavior and behavior change, including using technology to better understand and improve health, adherence, the mechanisms of behavior change, and behavioral interventions in complex patients in primary care. More specifically, her efforts in mobile and wireless health (mHealth) research include serving as the NIH lead for the NSF/NIH Smart and Connected Health announcement, convening meetings to address methodology in mobile technology research, serving on numerous federal mHealth initiatives, and leading the NIH mHealth training institutes. Dr. Nilsen is also the chair of the Adherence Network, a trans-NIH effort to enhance and develop the science of adherence. She is also a member of the Science of Behavior Change, Health Economics, and HMO (health maintenance organization) Collaboratory working groups. These projects are initiatives funded through the Common Fund that target behavioral and social sciences research to improve health across a wide range of domains. Dr. Nilsen also chairs the NIH Integrating Health Strategies workgroup that supports the science of behavioral treatments for patients with multiple chronic conditions in primary care. At NSF, she leads the Smart Health program, which targets science at the intersection between computer science, engineering, medicine, and health, broadly defined.

Cameron Norman is the principal of CENSE Research + Design and an adjunct professor in the Dalla Lana School of Public Health at the University of Toronto. Cameron's research interests focus on the intersection of systems science, design, and behavior science for health promotion and organizational change. The emphasis of his work is on program evaluation and modeling approaches to understanding complexity in social and health environments. Dr. Norman holds undergraduate and master's degrees in psychology and a doctorate in public health sciences from the University of Toronto, and completed a Canadian Institutes of Health Research postdoctoral fellowship in Systems Thinking and Knowledge Translation jointly at the University of British Columbia in Vancouver and the Centre for Global eHealth Innovation in Toronto. He recently completed a Master of Design in Strategic Foresight and Innovation at OCAD University.

Ruth Parker, M.D., is a professor of medicine at the Emory University School of Medicine. She is also associate director of the Faculty Development program in the Division of General Medicine, and holds a secondary appointment at Emory's Rollins School of Public Health. Over the past 15 years, Dr. Parker has focused extensively on health care issues of underserved populations, particularly health literacy. She helped create a widely used measurement tool to quantify patients' ability to read and understand health information. Dr. Parker currently serves as consultant and advisor to numerous federal agencies, professional societies, and members of industry on their initiatives related to health literacy.

Misha Pavel, Ph.D., is a professor of practice jointly appointed between the College of Computer and Information Sciences and the Bouvé College of Health Sciences at Northeastern University. Dr. Pavel came to Boston from the position of program director of Smart and Connected Health on a leave from Oregon Health and Science University where he was a professor at the Department of Biomedical Engineering, with a joint appointment in the Department of Medical Informatics and Clinical Epidemiology. He is also a visiting professor at Technical University of Tampere. Previously he served as chair of the Department of Biomedical Engineering (he founded in 2001) and as director of the Point of Care Laboratory, which focuses on unobtrusive monitoring, neurobehavioral assessment, and computational modeling in support of health care, with a particular focus on chronic disease and elder care. His earlier academic appointments included positions at New York University and Stanford University. In addition to his academic career, Professor Pavel was a member of the technical staff at Bell Laboratories in the early 1970s, where his research included network analysis and modeling, and later at AT&T Laboratories with a focus on mobile and Internet-based technologies. He taught a number of courses in statistics for behavioral research at Stanford University and Oregon Health & Science University. He was one of the founding members of Oregon Research Center for Aging and Technology and is a member of the nascent Consortium for Technology for Proactive Care at Northeastern University. He has a Ph.D. in experimental psychology from New York University, an M.S. in electrical engineering from Stanford University, and a B.S. in electrical engineering from the Polytechnic Institute of Brooklyn. Dr. Pavel is a senior member of the Institute of Electrical and Electronics Engineers (IEEE).

Brian Raymond, M.P.H., is a senior health policy consultant at the Kaiser Permanente Institute for Health Policy. Mr. Raymond analyzes emerging policy issues and supports the health policy decision-making process within Kaiser Permanente. His current areas of focus include eHealth technology to address health disparities, obesity prevention, and health in all policies.

In addition to policy analysis, Mr. Raymond manages projects and roundtable discussions to produce suggestions for health policy improvement. Mr. Raymond received a bachelor's degree in community health administration from the University of California, Davis, and a master's degree in public health from the University of California, Berkeley.

Hayley Thompson, Ph.D., M.S., is currently an associate professor in the Department of Oncology at Wayne State University School of Medicine and a Scientific Member of the Karmanos Cancer Institute, a National Cancer Institute–designated comprehensive cancer center. Dr. Thompson and several investigators in our cancer center are interested in health interventions using mobile devices/social media to reduce disparities. She was just awarded a new R01 grant (R01 HS022955), enrolling a population-based sample of approximately 1,230 African American and white breast, prostate, and colorectal cancer survivors to assess general eHealth activity and personal health history management to develop a software application prototype to facilitate access to digital cancer survivorship resources. Dr. Thompson also leads an American Cancer Society Research Scholar grant for testing an intervention to improve posttreatment resources using eHealth technologies to provide better support for Latina breast cancer survivors in southwest Detroit.

Kimberlydawn Wisdom, M.D., M.S., is the senior vice president of Community Health & Equity and Chief Wellness and Diversity Officer at Henry Ford Health System. She is a board-certified emergency medicine physician, the chair of the Gail and Lois Warden Endowment on Multicultural Health, and Michigan's and the nation's first state-level surgeon general. In 2012 she was appointed by President Obama to serve on the Advisory Group on Prevention, Health Promotion and Integrative and Public Health. Since 1987 she has been on the faculty of the University of Michigan (UM) Medical School's Department of Medical Education and adjunct professor in the UM School of Public Health. Dr. Wisdom founded the award-winning African American Initiative for Male Health Improvement (AIM–HI) and most recently, the Women Inspired Neighborhood (WIN) Network, which aims to improve access to health care and reduce infant mortality in neighborhoods in Detroit. Since 2008, she has chaired the Detroit Infant Mortality Reduction Task Force. In 2007, she founded a youth leadership development effort—Generation With Promise (GWP)—designed to equip youth to drive policy, environmental, and behavioral change in their school and community. GWP youth were featured on the cover of *Modern Healthcare* in June 2014. Dr. Wisdom is the recipient of numerous awards, has authored several peer-reviewed publications and book chapters, and appeared on national television, including ABC's *Nightline*, and has presented to audiences across the country and internationally.

Noam Ziv is a recognized thought leader, experienced system architect, and advisor to numerous startups in wireless communication and mobile health care fields, and is the founder and CEO of Kesembe Inc. Mr. Ziv is serving as a judge in both Nokia Sensing XPrize Challenge competitions, and as a technical advisor to XPrize in the Qualcomm Tricorder XPrize Competition. Noam worked at Qualcomm for 23 years. His leadership roles there included overall technical and system engineering lead for Qualcomm's cellular infrastructure development program, Technical liaison to Nortel, Alcatel, and the Electronic and Telecommunications Research Institute (ETRI), South Korea. Mr. Ziv was vice president of engineering leading Qualcomm's Corporate Research and Development software organization for over a decade. He made significant contributions to the design and implementation of software, hardware, systems, protocols, and custom silicon circuits (ASICs). Mr. Ziv is the inventor and architect of Qualcomm's 2net platform, and was an active contributor to multiple key technologies and products. Mr. Ziv was also a member of the original team that invented and implemented CDMA (Code-Division Multiple Access) cellular communication technology. Mr. Ziv earned a bachelor of science in computer engineering at the Technion (Israel Institute of Technology) and has been granted more than 20 patents.